T0067146

FIT FOR THE KINGDOM

Physical Fitness, Nutrition and Spirituality

PANDORA N. KINARD

authorHOUSE®

AuthorHouse™
1663 Liberty Drive
Bloomington, IN 47403
www.authorhouse.com
Phone: 1 (800) 839-8640

Published by AuthorHouse 05/18/2015

ISBN: 978-1-4969-6571-4 (sc)
ISBN: 978-1-4969-6572-1 (e)

Print information available on the last page.

Contents

For my daughter Ayva and all those who ever loved, supported and believed in me, from the bottom of my heart I Thank you.

Introduction

Fit For the Kingdom: Physical Fitness, Nutrition, and Spirituality

Keep alert and pray. Otherwise temptation
will overpower you. For though the spirit
is willing enough, the body is weak!
—Matthew 26:41

The struggle to lose weight, eat right, and do the things that make us healthy can be a difficult one. I know because I have been there, right where you might be now. I tried, and I gave up, tried again and gave up again. I wanted to eat right and exercise, but I just couldn't get with it.

What I didn't understand then was that the struggle that I was in involved a strategy formed by the devil long ago. It was his plan to keep me in bondage. The food was good, but I hated my body. The more I ate and stayed inactive, the more I hated myself. Not only did I hate myself, but I hated those around me who were thinner.

Food had overpowered me. It was the cause of my low self-esteem, and it was the cause of my hatred toward other women. It dictated how I spent my time, who I dated (I would only go out with a person if eating was part of the date), and it determined my level of happiness. Even when I set out to lose the weight, I had no idea how much I was being influenced and controlled by food.

Satan had used food as a way to set up strongholds in my mind that were preventing me from being the woman that God wanted me to be. Why? Because all my choices revolved around my self-image.

The food was not evil, but my overindulgence caused me to be in poor physical health, which gave me low self-esteem, leading me to devalue myself in every way possible, especially when it came to relationships. My personal self hatred led me to be with people who treated me poorly, which only served to deepen my low self-esteem. Do you see how Satan set me up? It's like a domino effect, so don't be fooled into thinking that your inability to do what you need to do to be healthy is an isolated problem. Satan can and will use food as a weapon, and this can have an effect on other areas of your life.

All of these issues had been getting in the way of my level of spirituality, and I didn't even know it. The devil had declared war, and his weapon of choice was food. If he could get me to slowly destroy myself by overeating (and later under eating) and get me to hate myself and others, he was in control.

In the year 2000, the Lord helped me win my battle against being overweight. In a year and half's time, I lost over eighty pounds. I went from a size 18/20 to wearing size 1 and 2, I was so happy that I decided to become a personal fitness trainer and a nutritional consultant, so I could help others.

What's different about this book? I'm going to give you the advice you need to help your body, wrapped in the word of God to help your soul. This is not just a battle involving conquering the bad habits of the flesh but it is a battle against the thoughts in the heart and the mind that wage war against of our attainment of physical fitness. In this book I will go over many important concepts that are necessary for you to understand and follow in order to reach your weight loss and/or personal fitness goals. Along the way, the word of God is used in two ways to motivate you to the next level of health in your life and as a point of reference that creates a spiritual framework for understanding the different concepts in physical fitness and nutrition that this book unfolds.

But before you move on, I think it's important for me to share the other side of my weight-loss story, what happened after I lost the weight (we know that Satan does not quit). You would think all would be well. I lost all of that weight, and now I could just live this happy slim-girl life, right? Wrong!

Once I lost the weight, I became obsessed with staying thin (now I was afraid of food).

It says in God's word that He does not give us a spirit of fear (2 Tim 1:7), but there I was, afraid to eat. I could not see that it wasn't the food, but how the devil was using it to control me. I ate healthfully, but I knew that I wouldn't even allow myself to enjoy the occasional treat because I was afraid of gaining weight again. Then came the bingeing. I was depriving myself for so long that when I did get a taste of something I really wanted, I ate way too much and then felt bad, and then the self hatred slipped right back in. To this day, I still struggle somewhat, but now I know what I'm up against. I have learned that "we do not wrestle against flesh and blood, but against principalities, against powers, against rulers of darkness of this age, against spiritual host of wickedness in the heavenly places" (Eph 6:12).

Satan and his kingdom are what we are up against, so it is important that as we strive to become healthier, we use "the sword of the Spirit, which is the word of God" (Eph 6:17) as the foundation and as our weapon to counteract the strategies that keep us neglecting our health issues, poor physical condition, and our bad eating habits. As you read and apply the knowledge know that you are not in this alone:

"I discipline my body and bring it into subjection, lest when I have preached to others, I myself have become disqualified" (I Corinthians 9:27).

Chapter 1

"The Spiritual Importance of Physical Health"

The Lord Cares About Our Bodies

*"Do you not know that you are God's temple
and that God's Spirit dwells in you?"*
(1Corithians 3:16)

The first step to moving into a healthy, more active lifestyle is to realize that how we treat our bodies matters to God. In fact in Leviticus 10, 11, and 13, The Lord gives all types of instructions about how the body should be taken care of. In Chapter 11, God gave the Israelites very specific instructions about what they should and should not eat. These foods were referred to as either clean or unclean. With the exception that God was holy and he wanted His people to be holy(Deut 14:1–21), there is no explanation as to why God declared certain things that the Israelites could eat in terms of the animals, as clean or unclean, either acceptable or not acceptable, to be used as food. It is possible to speculate that as our maker and creator, God was sharing with his people the foods best suitable for their bodies.

The point of highlighting this set of scriptures is not to condemn anyone who eats anything that God had prohibited in the commandments he gave to the Israelites through Moses. After all, the Apostle Paul made it clear that "those who think it is right to eat anything must not look down on those who won't, and those who won't eat certain foods must not condemn those who do, for God has accepted them" (Rom 14:3).

These scriptures are important to mention, because I believe that they provide a perfect illustration of God's "deep concern for the health of his people."[1]

Our overeating and under eating is definitely a concern of God's because they determine what we physically can and cannot do. And for many of us, they are leading us down a very slow path of death.

The journey of losing weight, eating healthy, and becoming more active for the Christian must begin with the basic understanding of how our bodies, souls, and spirits are affected by our unhealthy habits and how physically active we are. I believe that it is the desire of God for his people to be as healthy as possible, and to be in the best shape we possibly can.

I believe that having a Godly perspective about eating right and being physically fit helps us approach our weight loss and health goals on a more spiritual level. This helps us move beyond vanity and brings us to a place where the goal becomes to please the Lord by taking care of ourselves.

I also believe tackling the problem from a spiritual rather than just a physical perspective breaks the strongholds of the enemy that are acting to keep us in an unhealthy state. Under this perspective, we not only deal with the physical aspects, but we look at how our eating habits affect our soul (thoughts and emotions) and vise versa, leading us down a path of constant defeat. This perspective shows us how we unknowingly make our vessels less usable for the Lord's service by over- or under eating.

I don't know about anyone else, but my journey to lose weight left me feeling defeated, which just caused me to eat more. I was not happy, and my unhappiness with my body and all of the other different emotions, to a certain extent, affected my worship.

Because our bodies belong to God he cares about we take care of them. If we neglect to consider the damage being done to our bodies

---

[1] *The Word in Life Study Bible*, New King James Version (: Thomas Nelson, Inc, 1993), 209.

through our unhealthy eating habits, we are in essence putting ourselves first, instead of considering how the Lord feels.

The Lord is not only concerned about our spiritual health; He cares about our physical health as well. The body is the vessel that carries the spirit, and it's through the vessel that we carry out much of the work God has for us to do.

Romans 12:1 tells us to "present our bodies as a living and holy sacrifice to God."Webster's dictionary defines sacrifice as: "to offer up; consecrate, dedicate, devote; donate, give, yield." It may also mean to "lose, drop, forfeit."

In the profession of our faith, we resolved to offer up, consecrate, and devote ourselves and yield to God's will. In this, we forfeited our own authority (appetites, desires, and will) in order that we ourselves would become a sacrifice to God; this includes giving our bodies to be part of Christ. In I Corinthians 3:16–17 Paul says we (our bodies) are "the temple of God," and that the Spirit of God dwells within us. He also says that "if any man defile the temple of God, him shall God destroy; for the temple of God is holy, which ye are." The word "defile", Miaino in greek is translated in one form of the word as meaning to "to pollute" [2]As Christians, our bodies are the temple of God, and the temple of God is a holy place. Poor eating habits and physical inactivity causes pollution of the body, and in just the same way we would make sure the church building is clean and that people respect it as a holy sanctuary of God, it is in this same manner that we should treat our bodies as the living sanctuary of God. Think about it: if God said that whosoever defiles the temple, him shall he destroy, as believers we should take this as a serious indication that God feels very strongly about how we treat the bodies he gave to us. Though God works through our spirits, the body must also be able. The body is what gets us around to do God's work.

Jesus tells us that "though the spirit is willing enough, the body is weak" (Mk. 14:38).

---

[2] WE Vine: Vine Expository Dictionary of Old and New Testament Words Thomas Nelson Inc. 1997.

The Body /Soul /Spirit Connection

How much we feed the spirit determines how we think (the soul). Much of how we think determines most of what we do: in this case, the steps we take to become healthier through the proper nutrition and exercise. For the Christian, developing the state of mind that will allow for a physical transformation to take place begins with a spiritual motivation to care for the body. This spiritual motivation comes from the word of God. As the spirit is fed, the thoughts will change, and new thoughts lead to new behavior patterns. There are many scriptures in the Bible that when applied to different concepts of nutrition and exercise, can take on a whole new meaning that can cause changes in the way we think, giving us the ability to transform our bodies and become healthier people, through being empowered by God's word.

Body/Soul

The health of the body and soul are connected. Our soul is our will, emotions, and intellect. At 3John1:2 the Elder addressed his friend Gaius with this statement: "I pray that all is well with you and that your body is in health, as I know your soul is." Here, John the Elder, in his statement made a connection between the health of the soul (our will, intellect, and emotions) and the health the body. In general, what goes on in our soul; how we think, and what we feel, determines what we do, in this case, how we treat our bodies. If we therefore allow the soul to be directed by God, and we allow him to change the way we think about food and physical activity, we will then be able to become healthier people. Because when God is in control, the soul is well, and our soul under God's direction, can lead us so that the body can be well also.

But without yielding to God's direction in this area of struggle, we are bound to continue walking in accordance to our own unhealthy food eating habits, and irregular physical activity patterns. To do this knowing that it goes against the desire of God for us to be healthy, is to walk in a form of disobedience in that the lust for food and it's over consumption becomes the driving force behind our eating patterns and physical activity behaviors, as opposed to those that would lend itself to improving and not destroying the body- which is the Lord's temple.

In Proverbs 25:16 where it mentions how honey is good, but too much of it can make you sick, I think, is a perfect illustration of how too much food, can be a detriment to us. Team that up with a physically inactive lifestyle, and you have a recipe for multitude of physical aliments and conditions that God may never have intended for us to deal with; all of which place some level of physical limitation on us (unnecessarily). Now think about how these aliments and conditions can place limitations on the physical vessel, a vessel that God uses us to carry out his spiritual assignments in a physical world.

Further what we eat determines how we function. In the book of Daniel, we see that Daniel and his friends, who had been chosen from among the captives of Israel to serve in the king's court, rejected the rich wine and food that King Nebuchadnezzar had assigned for them to eat while they were in training.

They were aware of how unhealthy and unclean the diet was, and how it might affect their bodies. With the permission of the king's attendant, the boys followed the healthier diet they knew would be better for them. After just ten days they were stronger and healthier than all of the others. It then says that God gave these young men an "unusual aptitude for learning" (Dan. 1:12-17).

Here I believe that the word establishes a connection between what we eat and the effect it has not only how physically strong we are but also on how well we learn. The Hebrew boys were determined to maintain the level of nutrition they were instructed by God to follow, and for it, God caused them to excel both physically and intellectually.

I think we can agree that whatever we do for God and give to Him should always be our best. Therefore if the bibles urges to give our bodies to God as a living sacrifice, it is a worth wild endeavor to first meditate on and consider if the sacrifice is what it should be, and if not take some positive steps to make it better; Giving up bad eating habits and getting into better physical shape can help us to do just that! We don't want to just give a sacrifice we want it to be as the apostle Paul says at the end of the verse at Romans 12:1; "holy and acceptable". The key is that in giving the body to God we want it to be an acceptable sacrifice to him. In

Malachi 1:8 the Lord expresses his displeasure with less than acceptable sacrifices; in fact He says that it was evil to offer any less than the best.

To sum it all up, the body and soul connection being made here is that if we wholeheartedly embrace the view that the body is in fact God's temple, and develop a sincere desire to present God with an acceptable sacrifice of the body, it will help change how we treat the body; and this is clear- "So a man thinks, so he does"

Body /Spirit

Constant overeating is a work of the flesh, but self-control is one of the fruits of the Spirit (Galations 5:23; (each of which is a product of the way we think;, to think in the flesh or to think according to the spirit).

The spirit and the flesh are always at war (Galations 6:17), and in this particular war, the purpose of the enemy would be to have us to slowly destroy the body through our personal eating habits.

In the word God, it tells us that we, because of our salvation and the power that we have through Christ, are no longer obligated to do "what the sinful nature urges ... (and) if you keep on following it (we) will perish" (Romans 8:12). When God saved us, He released us from being slaves to the flesh and gave us the freedom to follow His Spirit. In other words we don't have to, if we don't want to, continue to be flesh directed and dominated by any sinful natures; including that which involves our relationship to food. If we want to live better, feel, better, and look better, we can.

There are therefore three things we should understand as we embark upon this journey of change and transformation. First physical fitness and proper nutrition has a significant place of importance in the lives of God's people, second being dominated by any flesh natures that hinder this area can places physical limitations on us that can have spiritual implications, and third our adversary the devil uses food and physical in activity as a weapon against us.

Physical fitness and proper nutrition have a significant place in the lives of God's people because a lack there of can lead to a number of health conditions such as heart attack, stroke, diabetes, high blood pressure, and obesity to name a few. All of these conditions have the potential to bring about premature death to the body. I'm sure you know this. I'm sure this is not new news to you. We have all, heard it all. So how come we can't change? Because the battle is not just physical it's spiritual: "We fight not against flesh and blood enemies, but spiritual principalities and rulers in high places" (Ephesians 6:12). Sometimes intellectual knowledge is not enough, and knowing does not always translate into doing. But we know these health conditions make the body less prepared to be physically used by God, so it's about time to do something about it. God is ready to do his part are you ready to do yours? If yes, then know this although we are made of flesh we don't have to be dominated by the flesh. Over and under eating, and consuming the wrong types of foods on a regular basis is a product of a flesh dominated outlook which is to eat as much as we want (or not enough) and push the idea of exercising to the back burner. These behaviors carry the capacity to place us under physical limitation, with the spiritual implications because the condition of the body determines our ability to withstand long periods of sitting, standing, walking, running, working, and other physical activities, all of which could be part of the physical aspect of what the Lord may be calling you to do. To persist in such behaviors indicates a lack of self -control. A lack thereof is the opposite of the self control mentioned as one of the fruits of the Spirit in Galations 5:23; and as with any area of our lives not being dominated by the Spirit but by the flesh (in this case to mean those natures that are biblically sinful and therefore ungodly), is bound to produce sin.

As humans we have all sorts of physical appetites that call for our attention, with eating being one of the most prevalent. That being the case, it is essential, that we gain control over any poor food habits that have the power to harm our physical bodies, and even worse send us to an early death; if for nothing more than to have a better vessel that is fit for the kingdom, with the side effect of feeling really great about ourselves as we break free bad eating patterns and physical inactivity. The apostle Paul said something I found very insightful, while not directly related to the topic of eating right and exercising, that showed how our flesh nature, can impact our level of spiritual connectedness. In addressing the church the Apostle Paul talked about how some had allowed their appetites (the flesh) to become their god. (Philippians 3:17–19). In like fashion if we are not careful our appetite for food can become like a god in the sense that the appetite for food (the flesh nature), dominates our lifestyle. If the appetite becomes god, this is sin. As a teen and into my young adulthood I had such a strong addiction to food that I was uninterested in any social event that did not involve food (before, during or after the event). Someone would call me up to do something or go somewhere and my first question was "When are we going to eat", and the second was "where are we going to eat". Food was totally in control of my social calendar. Dating went pretty much the same. How much I liked or disliked someone was very much determined by where we went to eat. My desire to eat (perfectly normal, as we do need to eat) became a sin when it started to rule my life, and have a negative impact. When we lack self-control in one area of our lives, it is virtually impossible that will not have a negative impact on other areas of our lives. In my case: my ability to bond and properly socialize with others.

It is true indeed that we because we are carrying out spiritual assignments in a physical world, and in physical bodies, It is with a strong conviction that I am therefore convinced that a strong spirit and a healthy and strong body go hand in hand. To revisit the scripture in Mark 14:38, we read that Jesus asked the disciples to go and keep watch while he prayed. They went because their spirits were willing, but because they were physically tired, they kept falling asleep. This scripture is a perfect illustration of how the physical condition of one's body can interfere with something the Lord would desire for them to do. Jesus wanted the disciples to pray, but their physical condition prevented them from following through on the Lord's request. I believe this provides the basis for understanding that it is important for us to take our physical selves, just as it is important to involve ourselves in every aspect of our spirituality. It seems that we have forgotten that our physical vessels are in fact a gift from God, and though we are spiritual beings, the fact yet remains that we are housed in physical bodies and have been placed in a physical world to carry out God's business.

So whether we like it or not, accept it or reject it, we cannot ignore the need to do the things we know will help the body to be healthy and strong, including among other things, eating right and getting regular exercise. Someone might be thinking "can't God do all things"? And "can't I do all things through God who strengthens me"? (Philippians 4:13)…If God needs me to do something physically demanding he will just give me the strength to do so". Yes it is true that the Divine is ultimately, and in all things our power source physically and spiritually, but that does not mean we don't have to do our part. We know that God's Spirit can fall on us in an instant allowing us to beat an entire army single handedly. It is certainly true that as the word says we can do all things through Christ who strengthens us, but I don't believe that it negates the importance of doing our part to keep the body physically healthy so that we are physically as well as spiritually prepared to render our service unto the Lord.

Before king David became king over Israel, he served as a Sheppard over his father's sheep and goats (I Samuel 17:34-37). In this position, David fought both lions, and bears, to protect his father's flock. David says in verse 35 ***"I go after it with a club and rescue the lamb from its mouth. If the animal turns on me, I catch it by the jaw and club it to death"***(NLT). Wow! What kind of physical strength David must have had in order to do this; lions and bears are big strong animals! But he also yet gives God credit at verse 37 as being the one who rescued him (God as the source). Nevertheless, David's physical strength enabled him grab the jaw of lions and bears and kill them. Now that's a strong man! I'm quite sure that wrestling with a lion or a bear takes a great deal of physical strength and ability. You and I may never have to do that (thank God!), but I believe the example of David speaks the fact that the condition of our vessels has its place of importance, in rendering our service unto Lord, along with our spiritual gifting.

Food Is a Tool Used by the Enemy to Keep Us in Bondage

This is true weather you're unhealthy or are bound by fear of eating one wrong thing: for the person who is struggling with being overweight, food may act as a comfort in times of emotional stress, but that comes with excessive weight gain, which can produce low self-esteem and/or self-hatred, two emotional issues that can perpetuate more emotional stress and overeating, turning them into a continuous cycle of bondage.

For the person who does eat healthfully, food can be used as a tool of bondage by means of the development of an unhealthy fear about gaining weight, causing an individual to be obsessed with how much they eat; to the point where they are afraid of the slightest indulgence. It's not bondage because the person has decided to eat healthy, it's a form of bondage because the desire to eat healthy is motivated not by one's love for self and the vessel that God has given, but by fear. The bible boldly proclaims that "God has not given us a spirit of fear but that of power, love, and a sound mind" (2Timothy 1:7) food is good and needful for the body to survive and nothing to be feared yet under such circumstance food in and of itself becomes an enemy. This can result in the development of eating disorders like anorexia and bulimia. At this point, life begins to revolve around being thin. Through my own personal journey of weight loss I have experienced both sides of the coin, not having an eating disorder, but the fear of gaining weight and therefore motivating me not to eat, and occasionally indulge. I'm not saying that all people who chose not to eat as much as the general population are operating out of fear, what I'm saying is that there are some people out there whose food bondage come in the form of fear of gaining weight.

In both cases, Satan to a certain extent has managed to cause food to become more of a central theme in our existence then it ought to be. Negative feelings and thoughts about ourselves that develop as a result of such bondage can become strongholds, patterns of thought that make us do things that are counter to what God would want and have for us to do; affecting our walk with the Lord in a variety of ways. It tells us in Proverbs 4:23 that the things that are in our hearts (thoughts, beliefs, and feelings) affect everything we do. It is very rare that we will struggle in one area in our life and it will have no impact on other areas. In this case our physical health almost always is connected to what we see happening or not happening in other areas of our lives.

Lest we get discouraged let's remember that Satan is humanity's adversary, and has the authority to do things according to the flesh; this ground belongs to him"[3]., he cannot control our spirit (Eph. 2:2). That is

---

[3] Juanita Bynum, *Matters of the Heart* (City of publication: Publisher, year published) 28–29.

why our adversary the devil works so hard to get us to be more so led by our flesh than God's Spirit. If the flesh via overeating or even in under eating is our vice the enemy will use it control us, that is why becoming fit for the kingdom also means praying and using God's word to help and guides us in to a better place of physical health. "For the weapons of our warfare are not carnal (of this world), but they are mighty in God for the pulling down of strongholds" (2Cor 10:4). Our single most important weapon against the enemy and his plan to destroy us through poor eating habits and physical inactivity, is to pray that the strong man of poor eating habits and physical inactivity be pull down in our lives; It is in prayer that we can surrender those habits to the authority of Christ. We have to literally cleanse ourselves spiritually and mentally from everything within us that has been holding us back from being as healthy and fit as we want to be. I know how the enemy can hinder us in this way because he did it to me. But God showed me that I'm not the only one.

Christian culture, involve many celebratory practices (especially in the Black communities- in which I was proudly born and raised.), that revolve around food. When I was a teenager, I was a regular partaker in many wonderful eating festivities, especially in between a morning and an evening church service where it was customary to serve food. And believed me, I enjoyed them. But God showed me through personal experience, that overeating and/or eating the wrong foods, especially before a service, takes our minds off the word being taught (the spiritual food) and focuses our attention on our stomachs and how tired we feel. Often times, I would be more focused on my stomach, or how tired I was than the word being given. It is a well known in the fitness and nutrition industry that over eating and/or eating the wrong foods can produce the desire for sleep not long after. Tiredness can be a definite distracter at a time when the Lord is trying to impart into our spirit. In this way Satan can use food to significantly reduce our level of spiritual attentiveness. The body is full, but the spirit is being starved. The same effect occurs when a person starves the body (with the exception of a fast, which God wants).

Take a moment to think about how eating has affected your level of attention in a service or at any other place or event where your level of attentiveness was vital. Or better yet, how about when not eating at all (except on occasions when fasting is the goal) your attention was affected. Loss of focus due to over- under eating, and/or eating the wrong foods may have caused vital information to slip right by you.

There are many foods that produce the effect of sleepiness when eaten in excess. This includes but is not limited to white rice, pasta, bread, and foods that are high in fat. Included in this category of items, is some of the foods I love the most: macaroni and cheese, fried chicken, stuffing, cakes. The foods themselves are not bad; they become bad when we overdo it.

As mentioned previously any part of our lives not controlled by the Holy Spirit will produce sin. Satan operates through our unhealthy eating and inactivity to keep us in a form of bondage. This type of bondage can affect our spiritual walk with God, as the enemy uses it to play on our self-esteem, and in small ways become less pleased with our body image. This issue definitely has the ability to cause us to deep down inside, to hate ourselves. When we hate ourselves, for this and any other reason, we can't really see ourselves as God see us. This is a form of bondage. God does not desire for us to be in any type of bondage, so if you want to be free, with God's help it's time to fight, and be free!

The good news is that God's power can free you. The Lord truly desires to set us free from all things that have us in captivity, even from things that have created any negative relationship we have formed with food. God's can "work in us giving us the desire and power to do what pleases Him" (Philippians 2:13). There is no doubt in my mind that being more physically activity and eating right please him because I believe it communicates to God that we appreciate, and value the body; the body that he took time to craft and put together perfectly!

How do we begin? Again the bible tells us at Ephesians 6:12 that we are not "fighting against the flesh and blood" but against Satan and his kingdom. Because of this, the Lords says to you today that if you confess the problem, ask for forgiveness for not taking care of the temple, which is the Lord's sacrifice and the temple of the Holy Spirit, the Lord will deliver you out of bondage.

Again to get the victory in this area we must allow this area of our lives to be under the direction of the Holy Spirit. This can be done through prayer and by allowing the word of God and his word to be the driving force behind the steps we take to fix the problem. Throughout this book, you will see God's word being laid as a foundation for every nutritional and physical fitness concept being taught.

I want to make it clear that The Lord is able to do all things, so I in no way am suggesting that being physically fit and eating healthy is a prerequisite for God to use us. What I am saying is that out of our of own love for God, and the knowledge that our physical health and what we eat matters to him, we should seek to please Him by doing all we can to eat better, and be more active. And that while poor eating habits and a lack of physical activity are known to have adverse physical affects it's also important to recognize and understand that because every part of us (body soul and spirit) is connected, our spiritual health can be adversely affected as well.

Matthew 18:18 states, "Whatever is bound in earth will be bound in heaven, and whatever is loosed on earth will be loosed in heaven. So let's do it together...." We bind unhealthy eating and physical inactivity, and through God's Spirit, we will lose the health that God wants for us.

Throughout the rest of the book, I will share with you some important concepts in physical fitness and nutrition that will help you today to begin eating right and becoming more active. This is your day to become fit for the kingdom, to transform your body into the ready, willing, and able vessel able to carry out God's work here on earth.

Chapter 2

Portion Control

But when the Holy Spirit controls our lives, he will
produce this kind of fruit in us: love, joy, peace, patience,
kindness, goodness, faithfulness, and self control.
—Gal 5:22–23)

In Galatians 5:22–23, the Lord is describing the type of persons we will be if his Spirit is in control. The Lord wants us to develop these types of characteristics in every area of our lives. In order to lose weight and reach other fitness goals, it is required most of all that the Spirit produce in us love, patience, faithfulness, and self-control.

Producing change along this journey requires that we love the Lord and understand that it is his will that we be strong and eat the right amount of food. It is love for God and his concern about bodies that can help us to develop the healthy amount of love for ourselves, so that we desire to nourish the body properly.

Learning how to control the portions of food we consume requires patience. Poor eating habits do not develop overnight but are the result of years of training that began when we were children. The good news is that small changes make a big difference. At this point, be less concerned about what you're eating and focus more on how much of it you are eating. In my fitness classes and with my gym clients, I always teach portion control as the first factor in losing weight and becoming healthier.

To see the changes we want, we must be faithful, meaning we must faithfully make the choice every day at every meal to eat the right amount of food. This can be achieved through using smaller plates, because the bigger the plate, the more food we tend to put on it. This can also be achieved by using section plates. I tell my clients to fill the bigger portion up with veggies and use the remaining sides for the meat and the starchy foods.

Self-control is extremely important especially in this area of living. It is so easy to indulge more then we should all the time. Just about every occasion in our society, in every culture, and in our churches is marked with celebration through consuming large quantities of food. When we want to celebrate something no matter what it is, we generally do it by either going out to eat or cooking a big meal.

Part of becoming who I am today, came down to just exercising self-control. My very first attempt at portion control began in college. I started out by eating prepackaged frozen meals. Even though these types of meals are high in sodium, and different types of preservatives not known as being good for the body, it was the first step in training my body how to be satisfied with just enough. Eating this way changed the way I felt about how much food I needed to consume. After awhile I began to become satisfied with eating enough and not more than that. Did I crave more? Yes, I did, but the Holy Spirit, through this action, had began to produce in me the level of self-control that would later allow me to adopt other healthy eating habits. After I graduated from college, I learned even more about why portion control is important. Through my friend Cynthia (a nutritional consultant and personal trainer), I learned among many other things, how the amount I ate affected my level of energy throughout the day and my body's ability to burn stored fat.

As stated in the previous chapter, Proverbs 4:23 says in essence that how a person thinks (what is in the heart) determines who they are. Learning how to control how much you eat is a major step in retraining your thoughts (which is part of the soul) in a way that will produce physical changes. This is the type of soul-body connection that will allow you to reach your goals.

The Purpose of Food

The purpose of food is to supply energy to the body and supply the body with the nutrients it needs to function. Without food the body cannot live very long. Food is calculated in calorie units.

The calorie is the unit of measure used to describe energy. In food, the term *calorie* is an expression of the potential energy that will be derived from eating a specified amount of a given food. Food is so wonderful!!! But it can also be a deadly weapon. The purpose of a thing determines how we use it. When we misuse food to satisfy the emptiness in our soul (depression, loneliness, sadness, or to be happy), or to have something to do when we are bored then we are in big trouble. Even when we use food to show love (as most moms do), we run the risk of exposing ourselves and the ones we love to heart disease, diabetes and obesity. Food is one of the easiest, low key ways to slowly kill ourselves and the ones we love if we are not careful and educated.

Portion Control

As we move through the day and as we sleep, the body is constantly giving off energy (burning calories). Weight gain occurs when food intake (calories) exceeds the amount of energy being used by the body. Weight gain is the result of the body taking the food that is not being used for energy and storing it for use at a later date. The problem we run into with eating too much is that the body never comes to a state where it needs to reach into its reserves. The extra calories, which is converted into fat, just sits there within the fat cells; and as we eat more, the reserves become larger and larger, causing the outwards appearance of weight gain. Imagine it as adding cotton to a pillow (weight gain), and taking it away (weight loss), the deflated pillow gets flatter and flatter as cotton is taken out. That's what happens to your body as it begins to use the fat stores for energy.

This is where exercise and portion control come in. If we can reduce the amount of calories being consumed, while at the same time increasing the body's activity level through exercise, weight loss can be achieved.

It is not necessary to starve the body to do this. In fact, starving the body only causes the body to store even more food in the form of fat(discussed in more detail in Chapter 4)

General Portion/ Serving-Size Guidelines

The nutrition and calorie needs of each person are different, depending on many different factors such as height, weight composition (amount of muscle versus fat in the body), age, activity level, occupation, medical history, gender, food likes and dislikes, goals, and so on. There are general guidelines that everyone can start following today in order to control the amount of food intake. This begins with an understanding of serving sizes and food labels.

Bread, Rice, Pasta, and Other Grains

A serving of bread = one slice or one half of a bagel.

Since we can't make a sandwich with one slice of bread, try Pepperidge Farm, Wonder brand, or Arnold's light breads. Two slices of these breads have the same amount of calories as one slice of regular wheat or white bread. In fact, with these breads, the serving size is three slices, so you can eat three slices, and it will still be fewer calories then if you eat two slices of regular bread.

A serving of rice = 1 cup (8 oz.). Some rice brands are 3/4 cup (6½ oz.).
A serving of old fashion oatmeal = ½ cup uncooked, makes 1 cup cooked. Instant oatmeal is o.k. but old fashion is better because it has more fiber.
A serving of cereal is = One cup, 3/4 cup or ½ cup (*please read the food label*)
A serving of any pasta= 2oz uncooked. = one cup cooked
**Note: it is a good rule of thumb to consume fewer carbohydrates at dinner. By having a ½ serving of a starch verse 1 full serving it can decrease the body's fat storing capacity because most people don't need starches at night when they will soon go to bed.

Most restaurants serve us at least four times these amounts. And we do the same when we cook at home.

Meat

In general, a serving of meat = 3ounces, or a portion of the size of the palm of your hand. The serving size for men is slightly higher about 4-6oz, depending on the fitness goal. Hormonal differences between males and females make it easier for males to consume and digest higher servings of protein than females. Remember that food is of no nutritional value to you if it goes undigested.

Oils and Butter

The serving size for most oils and butters is 1 to 2 tablespoons.

In general I recommend eating only 1 tablespoon, because of the high fat content of these foods. Fats are essential to our diet because they give us the feeling of being full. Never strive to cut them out completely because it will leave you feeling hungry, which can cause overeating later. One tablespoon of fat is more than enough in any meal.

A serving a oil = 1 tablespoon.
A serving of butter = 1tablespoon.
A serving of peanut butter = 2 tablespoons. The rule of thumb is to use only 1 tablespoon, because 2 tablespoons = 190 calories.
A serving of mayonnaise = 1 tablespoon, which is 100 calories. It is easy to add almost 300 calories to any sandwich by using too much mayo.
A serving of salad dressing = 2 tablespoons. This generally equals between 100 to 200 calories (10 to 25 grams of fat).

Watching Unnecessary Calories

Watching our consumption of liquid calories is just as important as learning to control portions. Liquid calories such as those found in soda, juice, and other soft drinks, can add up very quickly. For example, one serving of most beverages is 8 ounces (1 cup). Most people consume beverages that come in 12 to 20 ounces containers. The nutrition labels on these beverages list the amount of calories according to an 8-ounceserving. This means that the 20-ounce soda that reads it has 100 calories is only giving you the amount of calories for 8 ounces. Since a 20 ounce container of soda is equal to two and a half servings of soda, a person will consume 250 calories by drinking the whole bottle. Drinking a 20-ounce soda is the equivalent to eating two Hershey's candy bars. The average 20 ounce container of soda also has about 26 grams of sugar and about 30 grams of carbohydrates per serving Two and a half servings of soda contain 65 grams of sugar and 75 grams of carbohydrates. The general daily recommended intake of carbohydrates for the average adult is 300 grams a day. Wow! With just the soda alone we can consume almost 1/3 of our intake for the day. No wonder it's so easy to get extra calories that turn into fat.

When added to the consumption of a high-calorie meal, a person could easily consume about 1000 calories in one sitting without even realizing it, all of which if not used, for energy, will be converted into and stored as fat.

I would suggest opting for water, diet soda, diet ice teas, or pouring soda and juice into an 8-ounce glass and having only that.

Portion Control Tips

1. When possible, use section plates instead of regular plates. Place starch items in the small sections, and meat and veggies in the large section.

2. When having a large dinner with many starch choices (bread, rice, potatoes), choose the two you want the most and leave the rest alone. Fill the rest of your plate with veggies and a piece of meat (or 3 oz. if the meat is not in thigh and leg sections).

3. Order a kids meal at fast-food places, and get an extra-large diet soda (the liquid will fill you up).

4. Drink two to three cups of water before you eat. Again, the liquid will help you feel full faster.

5. Have sweets and chip snacks that come in individual single-serving-size packages. If you can, avoid buying the several-serving container. Sometimes the more we have in front of us, the more we eat. If you have to buy in bulk, it is worth the time to separate the snack according to the serving size listed on the package (here is where a food scale and measuring cup will come in handy) into little sandwich bags. Then when you are ready to munch, you are less likely to eat more than you should.

6. When dinning out, ask your server to bring out a take-home container when he/she brings your meal. Put half the food in the container to take home, and then eat the other half that is left on your plate.

7. Eat only 1 cup of the rice in Chinese food orders. Throw the rest out or share it with someone else.

8. If you eat any kind of breakfast sandwich (this includes bagels), eat one half, and replace the other half with an apple, orange, or plum.

9. Eat slower and chew your food. This gives the brain time to register that you have consumed enough food. When we eat too fast the brain does not have time to process this information and we might still feel hungry and eat more, when in reality we have already eaten enough.

Get this today:

Measuring cups and spoons

A small food scale (can be purchased at supermarkets and health food stores). This usually cost about eight dollars. It can be used to weigh meat and other foods that list serving sizes in weight.

Do this today:

Begin to drink at least a 32-ounce bottle of water a day. If you already do this, increase your water intake by 8ounces (1cup).

These first steps might be easy for some and challenging for others, but with asking God to help us make changes, we must remember that we have a responsibility to do what needs to be done so that those changes can come forth. Bestselling author Joyce Meyer (*Battlefield of the Mind, Winning the Battle of Your Mind*, 1995), put it best when she told us that we must:

"Always remember that if God gives you whatever you ask him for, there is a responsibility that goes along with the blessing. Lazy demons may attack your mind and your feelings, but you have the mind of Christ. You can certainly recognize the devil's deception and press past your feelings and do what is right. Asking for something is easy ... being responsible for it is the part that develops character. ... set your mind to do what is in front of you and do not run from anything because it is challenging."[4]

If this seems too hard or too much work for you, I ask you this: What can be better than doing something for you that will improve you? Aren't you worth it? Often times, we look to others to invest in us, and pour into us, and love us. And there is nothing wrong with that. But YOU have to put into this process what you want to get out of it.

---

[4] Joyce Meyer, *The Battle Field of the Mind, Winning the Battle in your Mind* (Warner Faith New York, 1995), 205.

Chapter 3

Let's Get Moving

This command I am giving you today is not too
difficult for you to understand or perform.
—Deuteronomy 30:11

The Right Attitude Goes a Long Way:

Many people shy away from eating right and being physically active because they think that it is too hard. And the truth is in the beginning your flesh is going to fight against you. Think of your body as a car that you have not started up in a long time. The car might take a little while to start, but after a while, it begins to run smoothly again, especially if you're putting the right fuel in the tank.

The mind-set of thinking that doing cardio is "just too hard" is an idea planted by Satan. "[T]he enemy tries to inject this phrase into people's minds to try to get them to give up"[5]. In her book, "Battle Field of the Mind", author Joyce Meyers points out ten "wilderness mentalities" (wrong mind-sets) that prevent us from accomplishing our goals, Out of the ten I want to focus on number 3- "it's just too hard". The Old Testament book of Exodus chronicles the beginning of the journey of God's people- the children of Israel out of the land of Egypt to the land He promised to them. On the journey they had to travel through the wilderness. I can't imagine that traveling through the wilderness was the most comfortable mode of travel. Nevertheless, it was the way they had to go. Terribly for the people, it was their way of thinking that turned an eleven-day trip into a forty-year journey of basically going in circles. When it comes to exercising many of us can't get motivated to do so because in our minds, we set a goal we want to achieve, but then we say to God, "Please make everything easy; I can't take it if things are too hard. It is this way of thinking that causes people to struggle with weight

---

[5] Ibid., 209.

and other health conditions for years; going around in circles, just as the children of Israel did. We simply have the wrong attitude.

When we stop thinking that something is too hard, it becomes easier to do. If we could develop the mind-set that exercise is not too hard, it won't be. The choice is yours- you can change your mind- set and move forward or remain in the wilderness of unhealthiness for the rest of your life. The end of the story is that their mind-set among other things caused a whole generation of the children of Israel to die in the wilderness and never see the Promised Land. I'm going to share with you some things that will lead you out the wilderness of physical inactivity, and in to the promise land of physical fitness.

Cardio…What's The Point?- The science of why we need increased movement

Doing cardio helps us burn calories so that we can lose body fat and it improves the functioning of the cardiovascular system (which includes the heart and lungs). Losing body fat involves the process of converting stored fat into energy. Fat is stored in the adipomis cell[6], also known as the fat cells.

In order for the fat stored in the fat cells to be used for energy, the body must have a need for the energy. This need is created through increasing the level of cardiovascular activity (and weight training, discussed in Chapter 5). The need for the fat energy must be enough to cause the body to metabolize large amounts of fat stored in the fat cells. It is this emptying out of the fat cells that causes the changes of the body's physical appearance. The fat cells remain; they just reduce in size because there is a reduction in the amount of fat being stored in them.

Fat is converted into energy through a chemical reaction that "breaks the bond between its basic elements."[7] In order for this process to be complete, the cell must be supplied with a sufficient amount of oxygen.

---

[6] UCSD study clarifies Insulin's Role in Blocking release of energy in patients with type II diabetes (Is this a magazine article? Need author, publisher, date).

[7] Fat Metabolism: www.weightlossforall.com/fat-metabolism.htm.

Oxygen completes the chemical reaction that allows fat to be converted into energy. Therefore "how much fat is burned during exercises depends on the ability of the cardiovascular system to deliver enough oxygen to the cells in a sufficient time."[8]

Cardiovascular activity makes the cardiovascular system stronger, thus increasing the body's ability to transport oxygen faster. The *"law of thermogenics"* tells us "you lose weight if you burn more calories than you eat"[9]

It is important to understand that losing weight should involve losing body fat only and not muscle. People who do not eat enough of the right kinds of food and/or do too much cardio may lose not only body fat, but valuable muscle tissue. How much muscle tissue we have is one of the factors that determine our *metabolic rate:* how fast we burn the calories we eat.

Our weight consists of both body fat and muscle tissue; anything that is not fat is considered muscle. Most people have more muscle than fat. The point of cardio for the goal of fitness is to lose the fat while retaining or adding muscle. Both those who are considered overweight and those who are considered of a low weight can have high body fat levels. The following chart provides the healthy level of body fat composition for males and female within different age groups:

---

[8]   Ibid.

[9]   Michael A. Clark and Rodney J. Corn, *NASM Optimum Performance Training for Fitness Professional* (National Academy of Sports Medicine, Calabasas, CA, 2001), 172.

MALE

Age	Risky	Excellent	Good	Fair	Poor	Very Poor
19-24	<6%	10.8%	14.9%	19.0%	23.3%	>23.3%
25-29		12.8%	16.5%	20.3%	24.4%	
30-34		14.5%	18.0%	21.5%	25.2%	
35-39		16.1%	19.4%	22.6%	26.1%	
40-44		17.5%	20.5%	23.6%	26.9%	
45-49		18.6%	21.5%	24.5%	27.6%	
50-54		19.8%	22.7%	25.6%	28.7%	
55-59		20.2%	23.2%	26.2%	29.3%	
60+		20.3%	23.5%	26.7%	29.8%	

FEMALE

Age	RISKY	EXCELLENT	GOOD	FAIR	POOR	VERY POOR
19-24	<9%	18.9%	22.1%	25.0%	29.6%	>29.6%
25-29		18.9%	22.0%	25.4%	29.8%	
30-34		19.7%	22.7%	26.4%	30.5%	
35-39		21.0%	24.0%	27.7%	31.5%	
40-44		22.6%	25.6%	29.3%	32.8%	
45-49		24.3%	27.3%	30.9%	34.1%	
50-54		26.6%	29.7%	33.1%	36.2%	
55-59		27.4%	30.7%	34.0%	37.3%	
60+		27.6%	31.0%	34.4%	38.0%	

Most fitness facilities offer body fat testing for free. This number is worth knowing since it will give you an idea of just where you are. The most important part of setting any fitness goal, is to know where you're starting from; only than can you properly asses where you want to go.

I know at this point you might be saying, "What's the point of knowing all of this?" The point is to raise your level of consciousness about how your body is actually losing weight. You already know that exercise leads to weight loss, and now you know why. Now when you go to work out, you know exactly what is going on in your body and understand why you must exert a certain level of physical activity to achieve results you are looking for.

This process mimics our walk with God in that, as we come to understand what God wants of us and why, it raises our level of consciousness of how we act, and what's going on as we move through life. The process of real deep down understanding is the vehicle by which knowing his word converts us so that we not only know God's word but we apply God's word.

The Routine

A cardio routine should consist of a warm-up to prepare the body for the activity, decreasing the likelihood of injury and premature fatigue (generally two to five minutes); the activity (performed eighteen to fifty-five minutes); and a cool-down (five to ten minutes). The cool-down "provides the body with a smooth transition from exercise back to a steady state of rest."[10] Intensity is important. As your body becomes more efficient you will need to increase the workout intensity to continue to see desire changes in your body. The easiest way to judge intensity is by taking your 10 second heart rate. The chart below shows us by age, and intensity level where your target exercise heart rate should be.

AGE	55% beginner	60%	70% intermediate	80%	85% Advanced
15	19	21	24	27	29
20	18	20	23	27	28
25	18	19	23	26	28
30	17	19	22	25	27
35	17	19	22	25	26
40	17	18	21	24	26
45	16	18	20	23	25
50	16	17	20	23	24
55	15	17	19	22	23
60	15	16	19	21	23
65	14	16	18	21	22
70	14	15	18	20	21
75	13	15	17	19	21
80	13	14	16	19	20

Use the following chart to find your TARGET HEART RATE (10 second count):

**The figures above are averages, so use them only as general guidelines."

---

[10] Ibid., 169.

Taking a closer look at the chart a person between the ages 25 and 30 as a beginner would want their heart rate at about 17-18 beats per second, when conducting a 10 second count. As the person advances the goal is to reach 27-28 beats per 10 seconds. To get the beats per minute the 10 second heart rate is then multiplied by 6. In this age group the beginner at a 55% target heart rate would be at 102 to 108 beats per minute, with a goal of exercising at an eventual intensity of 85% which would be 162-168 beats per minute, or more if one desired to go that far; take note that the more conditioned person will in general reach their exercise heart rate faster that those within their age group. Heart rate can be taken right underneath the palm of the hand with two fingers or with two fingers underneath the jaw bone at the upper portion of the side of the neck.

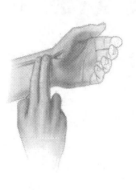 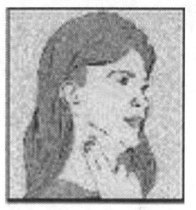

Burn More Calories in Less Time

The best way to burn more calories in less time, or in the same time, is to do interval intensity cardio training. Doing intensity cardio training helps to increase fitness levels, making it possible to burn more calories in less time. The overall goal is to progress by increasing the body's ability to work harder, in the same amount or less time, by manipulating different variables that make the activity harder (more intense).

The major strategy behind this method is do one to two minutes of moderate-intensity activity followed by a steady three to five minute increase of the speed, incline, or level of resistance, enough to make the activity high intensity (a level that makes it hard to speak and move at the same time). For example, on the treadmill, a person may start out by running at 4.5 miles per hour for two minutes, increase to 4.6, then 4.7, then 4.8, then 4.9, and then come back down to 4.6, for one to two minutes. This would be the pattern for the duration of the workout. On the last minute, the goal would be to sprint at a pace of 5.1 to 5.2, depending individual fitness levels.

For those who use cardio machines, I recommend starting at one to two levels or speeds below normal for the first two minutes of the workout as a warm-up, and then progressing at least two to four levels of speed, intensity, or resistance from the starting point. Once the high point is reached, speed or level should be reduced back down to one notch above the original starting point for one to two minutes.

For example, on the treadmill, manipulating for speed in a twenty-minute workout: Minutes

Speed	Minute- High Intensity Interval Cardio Training
3.0	1-2warm-up
3.1	3
3.2	4
3.3	5
3.4	6
3.5	7
3.2	8: Decease intensity and go back to speed
3.3	9
3.4	10
3.5	11
3.2	12
3.3	13
3.4	14
3.5	15
3.3	16
3.4	17
3.5	18
3.6	19
4.0	20: last minute 2-3 point speed level above where you were at minute 19

The same can be done on the elliptical machine and the bike by selecting the "random" or "interval" programs, and using the keypad to manipulate the level every minute in the same upward then down pattern. You can also stay within a certain rate per minute (RPM), which is displayed on the machine. Each week you can choose a different program on the machine (to vary that specific activity), and then every month, increase the level, speed, or both.

The intensity level of an aerobics class or video can be increased by using dumbbells and ankle weights. During kickboxing, I use ankle weights to create resistance while kicking and use 3 to 5 pound dumbbells to add some resistance to the punching movement. As long as the use of weight does not alter you ability to maintain the correct posture and motion pattern of the movements being performed, not only will this help you get a great cardio workout, but you can tone up and/or build muscle at the same time.

This method can also be applied to almost any outdoor activity as well, by choosing different running and hiking routes (some may be more hilly then others). For outdoor activities such as walking and running you can start out by waking one block, jogging one block, and then slowly increasing the amount blocks you jog before you run again. Or you can do a jog for 2 minutes, sprint for one. All the while you are doing the activity for the same amount of time.

It is important to increase the intensity at least once a month, or every four weeks. This means that the two-minute warm-up, the high point (the level or speed reached right before reducing the intensity), and the end point (last minute sprint) are increased by one notch, so whether your workout is twenty, thirty, or forty-five minutes, you never have to spend more time to achieve better results or blast through a weight-loss plateau. While the increases each month may be small, the body notices and will in turn burn 20 to 50 more calories per session then had been previously done. Before long, instead of burning only 100 to 200 calories per session, you'll burn 300 to 400 or more per session, in the same amount of time. In fact, those who normally spend more than thirty minutes doing cardio would experience increased calorie expenditure by decreasing the time and increasing the intensity of the session.

How Do I Know Where to Start?

It's all about making an honest assessment of what you feel level one through five is. You have to be able to say, "Hey, am I doing a level one amount of activity? Two?, three, four or five (five being close to the most intense you can do). Also use the target heart rate chart as a guide.

What Type of Cardio Should I Do?

Any form of activity walking, running, dancing, swimming, playing sports, or using cardio machines can be used as a form of cardio. The key is to get the heart rate elevated enough so that the activity is challenging enough to cause the desired changes.

Incorporating different types of activities into your routine is important for many reasons. First, each type of exercise will work the body in a different way, which allows the body to be constantly challenged. Challenging the many muscle groups in different ways through cardiovascular activity will make it less likely that the body will adapt to the point that you stop seeing the changes you want.

Adaptation is the process by which the body becomes so use to your routine that it takes less energy (calories burned) for you to perform the exercise than it did when you first started.

For example, although jogging and kickboxing may use the same muscle groups, they activate the muscles to work in totally different ways. So by including both as part my routine during the week my body is being challenged in more than one way. Some weeks I may not run or do kickboxing, but instead choose to do cardio classes for a week and then pick back up on the running. Or I may even use another type of cardio machine for a week, and then go back to my running. If you love to run like I do, or want to start a run program, take it from me- mix it up so to preserve your knees, back, and hips from injury.

It is also important to change your routine so that you don't get bored. Boredom is one of the leading causes why people abandon their cardio routine. If you are anything like me, you need some variety to keep it fun and enjoyable. So it's ok to deviate and try something else for a week or two. You can become fit and have fun too.

Cardio for Health versus Fitness

The National Academy of Sports Medicine Guidelines for Proper Integrated Cardio respiratory Training uses the "FITT" factors[11] as the underlying principles that one should consider when starting and maintaining a cardio regimen:

Frequency
Intensity
Time
Type

There is a "difference between the levels of activity required for health verses that necessary for increased fitness"[12] Consult with your physician before beginning any exercise regimen.

For general health:

Frequency	Intensity	Time	Type	Enjoyment
5–7 days a week	Moderate: enough to increase the heart rate and respiration	30 minutes total per day	General: walking using stairs mowing the yard	The higher, the better

---

[11] Ibid., 172.
[12] Ibid., 173.

For improved fitness:

Frequency	Intensity	Time	Type	Enjoyment
3–5 days a week	60–90 % of heart rate	20–60 minutes	Any activity	The higher, the better

Unless a person is training for a specific sport or training goal (like preparing for a marathon), I have found that it is unnecessary for the average person to spend more than twenty to forty-five minutes doing any cardio activity. The less time you spend doing the activity, the more intense you must make it. In other words, twenty-minute workout should be more intense then a thirty-minute workout, and so on and so forth. It's not as much about how long you spend doing cardio, as it is about how hard you are working while you are doing it.

The earthly ministry of the Lord Jesus Christ was only is said to have lasted for about all of three years, but in the time more was accomplished to reconcile humanity back to God, than had been done by any before him.

I use to spend an hour doing cardio every day to lose weight until I learned how to do more in less time. Now you can do the same.

Childhood Obesity- The importance of encouraging children to become physically activity

Train up a child in way he should go, and when
he grows old, he will not depart from it.
—Proverbs 22:6

Obesity in our society is as much of a problem in children as it in adults. In the United States, more than 13 percent of children between the ages of six and eleven, and 14 percent of adolescents twelve through nineteen are overweight.[13] And that number is continuing to increase. Children who are overweight have a higher risk of experiencing heart disease, high cholesterol, Type 2 diabetes, and high blood pressure than children who are not overweight. Overweight children have a 70 percent chance of becoming overweight adults. This percentage jumps up 10 percent if one or more of the parents are overweight or obese.[14] The problem of overweight children is a combination of lifestyle variables, such as lack of physical activity, poor eating habits, and genetics; lifestyle habits that allow for the full expression of any genetic predisposition toward obesity.

Sedentary activities that have become popular in our society for children and adolescents to engage in such as watching television, playing video games, and using the Internet as a form of entertainment has unquestionably contributed to the problem. About 43 percent of adolescents watch more then two hours of television every day.[15] On a positive note many video game companies have began creating more active dance and fitness games that get children moving.

Habits, especially our eating habits, are developed during childhood and usually carry over into adulthood. As parents, we try to raise our children the best way we know how, which is usually a reflection of how we ourselves were raised. Whatever we were taught gets passed on to our children (either consciously or subconsciously). Knowing this, it

---

[13] *Overweight in Children and Adolescents* www.mydna.com/health/weight/weightloss/obesity/overweight_child_teenhtml.

[14] Ibid., 2.

[15] Ibid., 2.

is important for parents to recognize that childhood obesity is mainly a product of the bad eating habits that our children pick up from us. The tragedy in this is that most parents don't understand this. They see their children gaining weight and/or eating the wrong foods, and chastise the child, when really they should be examining and chastising their own habits.

The word urges us to train a child in the way they should go and that the child when he/she is old will not depart from it. It is generally understood that this scripture refers to raising a child up in the things of God, but I believe that this scripture can be used to training that pertains to both the spiritual and the natural things, such as eating and physical activity habits. If children are raised up in the wrong things, it is possible that they will not depart from those things, either. When you think about it, children really have no say when it comes to making food selections; whatever a parent cooks or buys is what they have to eat. Parents who make bad food choices and/or overfeed their children can expect noting less then a child who will eventually grow up to eat more than he or she should and/or eat all the wrong things all the time. Parents, if you love your children, it's time that you take responsibility for your actions and begin to deal with your own bad eating habits first. Parents must not only tell their children how to eat right and be physically active, but they must show them how as well. Children need to see the principles of healthy eating and regular physical activity in action. In other words parents- don't talk about, be about it.

As an overweight child, and the daughter of an overweight mother I can testify to the fact that both parents and other family members unknowingly influence how you eat. Parents, especially mothers, often want children to eat everything that is cooked, and expect children to finish everything off their plates. In my family fried foods were staples and meals loaded with starches and laced with butter and salt were the order of the day. But as I entered my teen years, eating this way began to manifest into a weight problem. It was at this point I began to hear comments that I ate too much and I needed to "slow down." They didn't realize it, but it was unrealistic for them to expect me to change just to change. For children who are overweight the most immediate consequence is social discrimination and ridicule by both peers and family, which causes low self-esteem and depression. Ridicule from family is what I dealt with the most. They were unaware of how much many of their seemly passive comments and jokes were really affecting how I felt about myself on the inside. I'm sharing this to make parents more aware of how comments regarding their children's eating habits can damage children if not done in a loving and sensitive way. If you are not sure how to help your child about a weight problem seek the advice of someone who can. The time and effort you spend doing this can make all the difference in breaking or making your child.

Ephesians 4:4 warns us to be careful about how we joke around. It also says in the word that the "death and life are in the power of the tongue" (Proverbs 18:21) and that it is an "unruly evil, full of deadly poison" (James 3:8), so parents beware how you address this issue with your children. It is important to be sensitive about this issue; what seems like joking to you, may be driving your child into depression and low self-esteem. Putting them down doesn't work. Changing your own lifestyle and getting them involved in physical activity in a loving way does. It is also important to address siblings or other children in the home who ridicule an overweight child. If you are not sure how to do this in a constructive way that will teach the child doing the taunting a valuable lesson, use Christian literature and books that address this.

You can start out by letting your child know how much you love him or her, no matter what his or her weight is, by you as a parent [s] and by God. Your child probably already knows that he or she has a weight problem. Psalms 139:14 is a great scripture to share with them because it shows how David rejoiced about how wonderful his body was because it was created by God. It is important to allow your focus as a parent to be on your "child's health and their positive qualities, not on your child's weight"[16]-attack the problem, not the person.

Helping an overweight child is a family affair that involves gradual increases in the level of family physical activity and changes in eating habits. If your children see you eating and enjoying healthy food and physical activity, they are more likely to do the same and develop life-long habits.

---

[16] Ibid., 3.

If you believe your child has a weight problem, it is important to talk to a physician, who can make an official determination. It is important to talk to your child's doctor before making any changes to insure that his or her weight problem is not being caused by any underlying medical conditions.

Physical Activity and Healthy Eating Suggestions for children[17]

The "appropriate goal for most overweight children is to maintain their current weight while growing normally in height."[18] The goal for most children who are overweight and still growing is not to lose weight but to slow down the rate of weight gain so "they can grow into their weight." And any weight management program should be supervised by a physician.

Sixty minutes of moderate physical activity four to six days a week is the recommended amount of activity any child should have.

Getting children involved in sports and planning family activities that provide exercise and enjoyment for the whole family is important regardless of the weight of members in the family, because even normal-weight children and adults need physical activity to keep the body healthy.

Also, get the kids off the couch and into a playground or provide them and their friends with a safe environment where they can swim, bike, skate, play ball, or do other fun activities.

With regards to getting children to eat healthy many of the same rules apply that do for adults trying to eat more healthfully in addition to the following:

- First, your child's diet should be safe and nutritious and should include the daily recommended allowances of vitamins and minerals. One of the ways this can be achieved is through giving

---

[17] Ibid., 4.
[18] Ibid., 4.

your child a children's formula multivitamin. His or her doctor can suggest what might be best.

• Guide you family's food choices rather than dictate them.

• Encourage children to eat when hungry and to eat slowly.

• As much as possible, eat meals as a family, so they can see your choices.

• Carefully cut down on the amount of calories and fat in your family's diet.

• Don't place children on a restrictive diet.

• Avoid using food as a reward.

• Avoid withholding food as a punishment.

• Encourage children to drink water, and limit the amount of sodas and other soft drinks.

• Stock the fridge with low-fat and fat-free milk, fresh fruit, and veggies.

• Plan healthy snacks.

• Discourage eating meals while watching TV.

Finally support physical education curriculum in schools. A well-rounded physical education program offers your child an opportunity to be exposed to all types of physical activity, while educating them in concepts that will help develop the skills necessary to adopt physical fitness as a lifestyle.

As you can see, cardio does have a point. The point is to live and not die, the point is to feel better about yourself, the point is to cherish the body that God gave you by taking care of it, the point is to improve the health of our children- I could really go on; but I but think that you get it.

Today:

- Take the stairs instead of the elevator

- Park your car further and walk the distance

- Get up 10 minutes early and jog or do some jumping jacks

- Run around the park chasing your children or pet dog

- Bike to work

- Push the cart to the Laundromat, instead of driving

- Join the gym

- Get with some friends and do a workout tape together, and do it anyway if they don't come.

- Get some new workout gear to motivate you.

- Go up a speed or interval level on the treadmill, or your machine of choice.

- Try a new class

- Do some crunches and pushups during the commercials.

- Have fun doing cardio!! It's improving you

Chapter 4

Myths and Why Starvation Diets Don't Work

"Cry out for insight and understanding. …
for the Lord grants wisdom … [and] he grants
a treasure of good sense to the godly."
Proverbs 2: 3, 6, 7 [19]

Nutritional myths are the equivalent of strongholds planted by Satan in the form of information. Prayer and the right type of information, when accepted, have the ability to break down strongholds. My overweight condition caused me to pray for God's help. The Holy Spirit guided me to the right information, and when I accepted and applied what was being given to me, all the myths about losing weight and being healthy came crashing down. This process still continues in my life today.

Because there is so much information regarding nutrition and weight loss, the average person has a hard time figuring out what to do. As a certified fitness trainer, I too find it hard to keep up with all of the different fitness and nutrition fads and trends. Many of these fads and trends are dangerous and promote unhealthy eating extremes, and they are more myth-based than fact-based. The key to moving on from this point is to dispel some of the most commonly held myths about how to eat, what to eat, and when to eat. Doing so will better enable you to "Look straight ahead, and fix your eyes on what lies before you. Mark out a strait path and stay safe" (Prov 4:25-26).[20] My goal is to help you get to the truth so that you can reach and maintain your fitness and nutritional goals.

---

[19] *New Living Translation Bible* (Carol Stream, Illinois, Tyndale Publishers Inc, 2004), 531–532.

[20] Ibid., 533.

Common Myths

Carbohydrates Will Make Me Fat

The truth is that anytime you eat more calories than you burn, those extra calories will be stored as fat; whether they come from carbohydrates, fat, or protein.

Cut Out All Fat

Fat intake should never be below 10 percent of daily caloric intake, for several reasons. A certain amount of fat is necessary in each meal to provide a level of satisfaction so that hunger does not come back too soon. This can create the potential for overeating in subsequent meals. Fat plays a vital role in many body functions such as digestion and excretion. Some fats are good for you, like Omega 3 and 6 fatty acids found in fish, flaxseed oil, and other mono- and polyunsaturated fats.

Eating Fat Will Make You Fat

When the amount of calories taken in exceeds what is burned, weight gain will occur. With high-fat diets, it is easier for more to be consumed than what is really needed, because diets high in fat provide a lot more calories for a small volume (9 calories per gram of fat versus 4 calories per gram of carbohydrate or protein). Most people would find it hard to feel full eating only a small amount of food that is higher in fat. Think about how many cookies you would have to eat to get the same amount of fullness a healthy sandwich with some lean meat would provide.

Excess Calories Make You Fat, Not Eating Fat

It is important to understand that a diet low in saturated fat and very low in trans fats is one of the keys to losing and maintaining weight loss. But don't avoid fats altogether. Use mono- and polyunsaturated fats, which are good fats found in foods like olive oil, avocados, walnuts, tofu, and seafood.

A major reason why poly- and monounsaturated fats are considered good fats is that these fats melt at a lower room temperature than saturated and trans fats. With regards to losing and maintaining weight, this means that we don't have to produce as much energy (elevation in body temperature due to exercise and other activities), in order to burn the calories that come from these types of fats. Saturated and trans fats melt at significantly higher room temperatures, which means that it takes a lot more work (energy expenditure on our parts), to burn off the calories from these fats.

Trans fats are our new worst enemy in the battle to stave off excess weight. Trans fats are found mainly in processed foods and are not always listed in the fat content of food labels but within the ingredients. A trans fat is a mixture of fats and oils that are hydrogenated (combined) as a way to extend the shelf life of food. Trans fats are more dangerous than saturated fats because they raise cholesterol levels significantly higher than saturated fats do, and they can contribute to higher levels of weight gain, making it hard to lose or maintain weight.

Currently, the Food and Drug Administration (FDA) does not require that food manufacturers list trans fats as part of the fat content on nutritional labels. The amount of trans fats in a product generally increase the fat content in many products by 3 grams or more. As a result, many products marketed as fat-free or low-fat may in fact contain high levels of fat that its makers are not required to report to us; so buyer beware! Look in the ingredients, if you see the words "partially hydrogenated" anywhere within the ingredients, the products contains trans fats. Also, the closer those words appear to the top of the ingredient list the more trans fat it contains. Food manufactures list food ingredients from greatest to least.

What Is Insulin's Role in Storing Fat?

After eating a meal, insulin is secreted and is responsible for the storage of glucose and amino acids (the "energy" produced from the breakdown of food). This energy is released throughout the day to fuel all of our activities. Fat is the primary fuel source the body uses during normal activity. As insulin levels begin to decrease, the hormone glycogen takes over, and it's release tells the body to continue to release stored fat, because for that time no new food energy sources are coming in.

If too many calories are being consumed, the body is still releasing that fat energy, but the body is never at a point where what is being released is making a difference in lowering weight because there is so much of it being stored. Insulin is only a mechanism for storing fat. The amount of calories we eat cause fat stores to increase.

Before food can be used as energy, it is broken down into a simple sugar called glucose (which is what occurs during digestion). When the glucose enters the blood, it stimulates the production of insulin. Insulin acts as the vehicle that delivers glucose into the cells. Extra glucose (energy) is stored in the form of fat in fat cells. Very high levels of glucose in the blood (the result of overeating), simulate the production of very high levels of insulin, the hormone vehicle by which energy is stored as fat in the fat cells of the body.

Another important hormone that is connected to fat storage is the hormone citosol. This hormone responds to high levels of stress by causing the body to store fat. Citosol is at its highest when insulin levels are high. When the levels of citosol and insulin are high, the levels of glycogen are low. When this happens we are more likely to store calories as fat. The key to controlling our insulin and citosol levels is to eat five to six small meals a day (which we will cover in Chapter 8), and to regularly choose foods that don't cause enormous spikes in insulin production after consumed (discussed in Chapter 6).

White breads, white rice, and white pastas are foods that usually trigger this reaction. This does not mean you have to give these foods up completely, but they must be consumed in moderation by eating no more than the serving size. But realize as highlighted in Chapter 2, that these particular foods are not as filling as whole grain products because of the general lack of sufficient amount of fiber. Without fiber which is very filling, many people fail to feel full from just a serving, and will usually overeat.

Eating After 7:00 PM Especially Carbs) Causes Weight Gain

Your body does not have a clock that says, "OK, after seven, let's store carbs as fat." If you have to eat later in the day because of changes in your schedule, gaining weight is not an issue as long as you are not consuming more than what your daily caloric intake should be. The best thing to do is to spread calories evenly throughout the day to avoid energy dips that may make you crave more. This is done by eating five to six small meals every three hours: three main meals and two to three snacks.

Losing Fat and Gaining Lean Muscle Requires a High- Protein Diet

Too much protein and not enough fat and carbohydrates will cause the body to use protein as a primary energy source instead of the fat or carbohydrates. When this occurs, very little of the protein compounds are being used to build muscle. This can result in no gain at all, and even worse, a loss of muscle. A lost of muscle will result in a decrease in one's metabolism because muscle uses about four times the amount of energy to maintain itself than fat does.

Stick to Eating Three Meals a Day

The truth is that most people nibble in between meals anyway, so it is best to break the three meals up into five or six smaller meals (discussed in more detail in Chapter 8). Doing so will help keep the blood sugar (insulin) level stable, making it more likely that the food being consumed is more often burned than stored as fat. Making better food selections and watching portions are key component here.

Bad Genetics Cause Weight Gain

While it is true that a segment of the population has a hard time experiencing weight loss because of a genetic disposition, for the most part, excessive weight gain and obesity in our society results from "an environment of caloric abundance and relative physical inactivity that is modulated by a susceptible genotype."[21] In other words, the answer for the majority of people is not the gene alone, it is the interaction with other environmental factors, such as food intake and level of physical activity, that determine the degree to which any genetic predisposition to weight gain will be expressed. I'll use myself as a prime example.

---

[21] *Obesity and Genetics*, Center for Disease Control www.cdc.gov/genomics/ training/perspectives/files/obesedit.htm.

In my family, many of the women are overweight, meaning that for their height and weight they have a high level of body fat relative to their age. Most of the women, including myself, were overweight as children, so it is safe to say that in my family, there is more a genetic predisposition toward weight gain than not. But because I was successful at losing weight and keeping it off, I can say with 100 percent certainly that lifestyles, culture and, behavior are contributing factors to the weight problem in my family. Because I am aware of my genetic predisposition, I tend to put on weight a little easier (especially in the waistline), I therefore pay attention to what goes into my body and make sure I maintain a certain level of physical activity. My happy medium is between 120 and 125; 130 being the max. I realize my genetics do come into play regarding how physically developed I can become without the use of dangerous supplements that many who want that perfect physique use; so I have accepted that no matter what I do, I'll always have that little lower belly pouch, and that's fine. Even at my lowest weight of 112 pounds and totally muscular, I still had that little nagging pouch. But it was at that point that I just learned to accept it and move on, because I knew that I was at my optimal level of fitness.

Eating Very Little Will Cause Weight Loss

The body is an amazing structure that was designed by God to help us survive. Part of the innate survival mechanism of the body is the body's ability to work to fix system imbalances (such as the ones created when we don't eat enough food). When the body senses an imbalance, such as eating too little, it will slow down certain body functions so that it can preserve and devote more energy to other essential task. When this occurs, people begin to experience symptoms of problems they never had before. For example, when you don't get enough sleep, the brain doesn't function as well. You may feel forgetful and may be unable to think clearly. Therefore, deprivation leads to stagnation. Depriving the body of food causes it to slow down your metabolism (the rate at which you burn calories) in order to help you to survive.

In times of famine the body will do what it takes to preserve us from dying. One of the ways that the body does this is by going in what I like to call a power- save mode. In the same way that putting a computer on power save helps reduce the amount energy we use and can save us money, the body will reduce the amount of energy it uses by storing more calories as fat, when it thinks we are starving. The overall result in the end- is more weight gain than weight loss.

Starvation diets don't work for long. Drastically reducing calories causes the body to slow the rate at which it carries out bodily functions (including burning calories) because it thinks that you are starving. As part of the survival-starvation mode, the body will begin to burn less calories, and instead choose to store the calories as fat in order to preserve the individual. While in the short run weight loss can be achieved, in the long run you actually end up gaining weight— sometimes more then what you started with. This weight is often harder to lose because through the process of starvation, you have made the body less willing to burn the calories being consumed.

The other problem with eating too little is that in order to experience continual weight loss, you must continue to reduce how much you eat; which further reduces your metabolism by virtue of the body's preservation process.

It is important to understand that under eating, too, is a form of self-abuse. Any form of self-abuse is not acceptable to God. The scriptures say:

> *Or don't you know that your body is the temple of the*
> *Holy Spirit, who lives in you and was given to you by*
> *God? You do not belong to yourself. For God bought you*
> *with a high price. So you must honor him with your body.*
> (I Cor. 6:19–20).[22]

The Holy Spirit was given to help us in every area of our lives, so unlike the world, we have the power through God's Spirit to change.

From my own personal experience I know what it is like to be so desperate to lose weight that starving myself seemed to be the only answer. The end result was I would only end up pigging out. There goes Satan again. Either I was going to starve to death or eat myself to death, either way the enemy would win. After I would overeat, I would

---

[22] Ibid., 928.

feel so bad that sometimes I would make myself throw up. Food myths became strongholds in my mind that caused me to abuse my body by eating too little, and then eating too much, opening the doorway for the demons of anorexia and bulimia to come in. But thanks be to God, this cycle didn't last too long. For a while, I just gave up on to trying to eat right. But this only served to perpetuate another stronghold that I was never going to be able to change; the devil had me right where he wanted me. But God had other plans. He had me try again, but this time he was in charge. With him in charge, not only did I lose the weight and build muscle, he allowed me to use the very condition that had oppressed me to become a source of financial prosperity through becoming a personal fitness trainer. With the Lord in charge, what seemed to me to be a hopeless situation turned into a place where God blessed me with more then I had ever expected to gain. Peter experienced a similar situation.

In Luke 5:8–10,[23] Jesus was preaching to the masses near the Sea of Galilee and had asked Peter (who was called Simon and was not yet an apostle) to use his boat so that he could speak from the water. When the Lord was through teaching, he told Peter, "Now go out where it is deeper and let down your net, and you will catch many fish." Peter said to the Lord, "Master, we worked all night and didn't catch a thing, But if you say so, we will try again," and when he did, they caught so many fish that the boat begin to sink. Peter had tried all night to catch fish and was unsuccessful, but at the Lord's urging, he tried again. he doubted himself but trusted the Lord. With the Lord in charge this time, he tried again; and the end result was overflow. So maybe you have tried to eat right and lose weight. Maybe you're just stuck at a plateau. In order to reach your goal, the Lord says to you today as he said to Peter, "You must go deeper." Deeper in prayer to war against those things that would seek to hinder you, deeper in your relationship with God, deeper in your ability to listen to the Holy Spirit who is our teacher and counselor, deeper in your understanding of God's word and the ability to use the word to draw strength to accomplish your goal, deeper in your quest to gain the right information, deeper in your effort to apply what you are learning, not tomorrow, but right now By doing so, God will tear down every stronghold that is telling you that you can't, believe. God says you can. God through his Spirit will direct you to the right information so that

---

[23] Ibid., 824.

you can reach your weight loss or fitness goal without harming your body. Remember that Satan has people everywhere, even in the nutrition and physical fitness industry; that's why there are so many people literally dying to be thin, and/or put so much pressure on themselves to look a certain way.

Before going on to the next chapter, pray this prayer:

Father in the name of Jesus, I ask that you tear down every
stronghold that has been created through misinformation
about how to eat properly. In Jesus name, I
forbid any seeds of misinformation
to be planted that would cause me to harm my
body in any way. I ask you, Father, to close any
demonic doorways that have been opened because
I believed such information. Lord, I thank you that from
now on, I will call on the Holy Spirit to expose to me the lies of
Satan in this area. Lord, I am committed to learning how to
eat through the right type of information, which I
am trusting you right now to lead me to. By my faith in you,
I count it as done, and I thank you. In Jesus name, I pray.
Amen

Chapter 5

Strength Training

Zeal without knowledge is not good a person who
moves too quickly may go the wrong way.
—Proverbs 19:2

One of the biggest spiritual revelations that I have had in my life is that strength training is similar to spiritual training. When I first gave my life over to Christ, I didn't know what to do or what to expect. All I knew was that God loved me and I wanted to be right with him, but I strayed away for a while because I had a lot of enthusiasm but no direction. I had the information (the Bible), but I didn't know how to make sense of God's word enough to apply it. I had a similar experience when I decided to lose weight and start strength training. I was so happy that I had finally made the decision to do it, but like most, I didn't have clue where to start or what to do and for a while I just did whatever. There was a lot of information available about strength training, but I didn't know how to apply the concepts to myself. It was the same way with my walk with God. Once I started seeking wise counsel concerning the things of God, I began to practice what I was being taught. The more and more I practiced implementing the word of God in my life, the stronger my spirit became, and is still becoming.

Similarly, with strength training, by being diligent and consistent, I was able to build a strong body. With each repetition you do, your muscles get stronger, and over time you will experience a change. This is an important parallel between spirituality and strength training. Spiritually, while God is helping you to get rid of the ways of thinking and situations that cause us to be unhealthy, we need to build up the strength in this area in our mind that was once full of the wrong ideas with the right ones. Each time you practice what you have learned, you become spiritually stronger. This growth has the ability to cause changes. The changes that we experience spiritually (through the word), which produce changes mentally (how we think), can only be maintained through the repetition of regular training. As we do so, our ability to walk closely with God and to understand what he requires of us in this and any other areas of our lives becomes deeper.

In the Natural

Once you lose weight, strength training helps to tighten and tone so that you will not be flabby. Also, strength training helps to build muscle, which helps speed up your metabolism, increasing your ability to burn calories. The more muscle you have, the more, food you can eat, because muscle tissue needs more calories to maintain itself than do fat tissues. Also doing cardiovascular training, absent of strength training, may cause a breakdown in the muscle tissue.

Getting the right type of routine and learning how to create variety and progress is very important, but it is even more important to understand different concepts of strength training. Understanding these concepts will make you less likely to make mistakes, get bored, and/or do the wrong type of exercises. It is also important to seek the advice of a doctor before starting any type of strength training routine, especially if you have any preexisting medical conditions, or are on medications that cause fatigue, have a history of any type of back pain, or have had any type of major surgery. These conditions will determine what is and what is not safe for you to do. Also enlisting the help of a personal fitness trainer could also be beneficial.

Benefits of Strength Training[24]

Strength training:

- Improves cardiovascular efficiency

- Increases lean muscle body mass

- Decreases body fat

- Increases metabolism

- Increases bone density

Beyond improving your health, the appearance of your body, and making you feel good (which you will), strength training can better prepare you to be used by God physically. For example, many preachers and evangelists find themselves standing for long periods of time. It helps to have strong legs. This is only one of many reason why strength training can be is important for those who carry out the work of God.

Vocabulary

Strength training is the process by which the muscles (under the control of the nervous system) "generate internal tension that manipulates the bones of our body to produce movement" and "exert resistance against an external force."[25]

A *rep* (short for repetitions) is the single action of lifting the weight from the start to the finish position during a weight-training exercise.

A *set* is performing a specific number of reps at one time without resting in between. For example, repeating a bicep curl ten times, resting, then doing it again. Each group of ten represents a set.

---

[24] Michael A. Clark, and Rodney J. Corn, *Optimum Performance Training* (Chandler, Arizona; National Academy of Sports Training, 2004),15 and 241.

[25] Ibid pg230

Types of Strength Training[26]

There are various types of strength training that fit into the general categories below. Exercise selection with each category depends on individual health, fitness, and/or sports goals. The concept of specificity is that the selection of a specific strength training activity is based specifically upon the muscle being trained, and why. The difficulty most people have with getting into the habit of strength training is that they don't know what to do, or have little understanding as to why it is important to train the body a certain way. Most people just do what they see others do, and sometimes that person is either training in a way that may not be suitable for your specific needs or they of doing it all wrong. It is not always wise to follow what others are doing, but invest some time in finding out and doing what works for you.

Types	Purpose
Speed strength	Developing the ability of the muscles to move quickly in a short period of time. For example, to swing a bat.
Endurance strength	Developing the ability of the muscles to sustain long periods of activity. For example, running a marathon.
Stabilization strength	Developing the ability of the muscles to maintain the body's balance during movement.
Core strength	Developing the muscles of the lower back, hips, and the midsection to improve the body's ability to control an individual's

All of these forms of strength not only exist in the natural world, but they exist in the spiritual world as well. In our walk with God, we need

---

[26] Ibid pg241

the strength to move quickly (immediately obey the voice of God no matter what He's telling us to do, and not drag our feet). We also need to develop the strength to endure all things. Understanding and applying God's word can help us to develop a level of spiritual stability that allows us to maintain our balance and not fall off spiritually, mentally, emotionally, or physically as we move through life. Core strength is developed in us as we allow God to strengthen the weak innermost parts of our heart through our spirit, which is done by accepting and applying the word of God. The spirit is the core of our being; if the core is not strong, we will find ourselves constantly succumbing to temptation and being deceived by the devil. Functional strength can be developed as we allow God to use us in any way He sees fit, meaning you being open to him. As we allow Him to use us, we become more functional vessels in many areas. As we do so, we can come to have a personal knowledge and understanding of the power of God. Finally, if we put all our trust in God and lean not on our own understanding, (Proverb 3:4) He will develop in us the strength to operate at the ideal level needed to carry out our functional activities for the kingdom.

The Major Muscle Groups

Unless you are a body builder, a fitness competitor, of an athlete, there is really no reason to over complicate your weight training routine. If you focus on training the major muscle groups of the upper, middle, and lower body, you will do just fine.

The muscles of the upper body include:

- Back

- Chest

- Shoulders

- Biceps

- Triceps

Generally the goal is to train both the upper and lower body at least twice a week.

The muscle groups of midsection include:

- The *rectus abdominis* muscles: the front of the midsection from the lower chest to the pubic bone, aka, the six pack. They can be trained by properly performing crunches and other ab exercises.

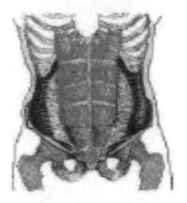

- The *obliques*: the muscles that run alongside the midsection from the lower rib cage to the pubic area. These muscles help your torso flex to the side, twist, and bend forward. They can be properly trained by doing side bends and side crunches.

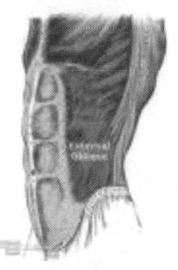

- The *transverse abdominis* this muscle runs across the abdomen and helps keep the internal organs in place. It forces out breath (like when doing a crunch) and helps to stabilize the spine. It can be properly trained by pushing all of the air out of the stomach during a crunch or by twisting from side to side.

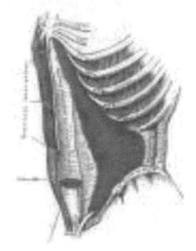

- The *erector spine:* a pair of muscles that run along the side of the spine. These muscles keep the spine erect and allow twisting to take place. They can be trained by properly bending forward from a standing position with or without weight.

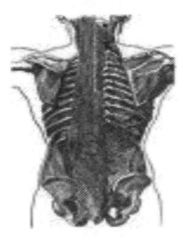

I though it important to include these photos of the different parts of the mid section also known as the core so that during your training time you will understand that there different exercises that target each one of the core muscle groups. The majority of people focus primarily on the rectus abdominals, and the oblique. So that all muscles get the fair treatment it might be helpful to focus on two groups per work-out, or do 1 to 2 sets of an exercise for each muscle group. It might take anywhere from 10-15minutes to do this, so plan for it.

The muscles of the lower body include:

*   The quadriceps (front of the leg)

*   the hamstrings (the back of the leg)

*   The gluteus maximus, minimus, medius and med (the butt)

*   the calves

*   The inner and outer thigh
    The best way to train these muscles really depends on the individual goal. In general slow controlled movements with at least a 2 second squeeze to tighten the muscles while performing the selected strength training activity, I believe create a good quality of motion that provide optimal results.

How Should I Work Out?

No matter if you're in the gym or at home (discussed further later), there is a certain amount of reps and sets that you need to do depending on your goal.

Resistance Training Systems[27]

Type	Definition
Single-set system	Performing one set of each exercise. For example, one set of bicep curls.
Multiple- set system	Doing more then one set of each exercise.
Pyramid system	Increasing the weight with each set or decreasing the weight with each set.
Superset system	Performing a couple of exercises in rapid succession of one another. For example, performing a set of leg extensions and then performing a set doing squats.
Circuit-training system	Performing a series of three or more exercises one after another with minimal rest.
Split-routine system	Performing a routine that addresses the various parts of the body to be trained on separate days.

In my personal routine, I combine the pyramid, superset, and split-routine method by Increasing or decreasing my weight with each set, performing two exercises for each body part in rapid succession of one another, by training my upper body one day, and my lower body another day. Sometimes I circuit train as well because the continuous movement elevates my heart rate, helping me to burn more calories during the workout. I also may do all front of the body muscles one day (chest

---

[27] Ibid., 241.

biceps, abs-including the oblique, quads and, shoulders) one day, and do the muscles in the back of my body (shoulders, back, erector spine, hamstrings, gluteus-the butt, and calves) on another day, just to do something different. When I'm really short on time in a given week I will mix cardio in with my weight training. I will do let's say upper body, and after I work each body part for 6 sets I will jump on the treadmill for 3-5minutes, each time I get on the treadmill, I increase the speed anywhere from 1-5 levels. All together this takes me about 45minuts, and I'm done. I get at least 25minutes of cardio out of this. But you better to believe it is intense!!

Increasing muscle size vs. Improving muscle tightness

If your goal is to increase the size of the muscle, then in your strength training routine you will perform fewer repetitions at a higher weight. The rep range will be between 6-12, at a weight where at about the second to the last rep you should feel your muscles ready to give up. Please remember that the weight you choose should also allow you to keep proper form and technique through the full range of motion of the exercise being performed.

If your goal if to increase muscle firmness, but not the size of the muscle, then in your strength training routine you will perform more repetitions at a lower weight. The rep rage will be 12 to 20 reps. The amount of weight being used should be enough that the muscles feel ready to fail at about the third to the last rep. so if you are doing 15 reps by rep number 13 the muscles should feel almost ready to give up. Again all exercise and weight selection should allow you to maintain proper form for the full range of motion, and for the duration of performing the exercise.

Improperly performing an exercise can lead to injury. It's better to be safe than sorry, as excited as we are about our journey to be fit for the kingdom, we must also exercise wisdom in how we do it. Remember this is a lifestyle change being made, not a passing fitness fad so lets take our time and do it right.

Training at Home

In October of 2004, I was hit by a truck while jogging one morning. By the grace of God, I didn't suffer any of the major injuries you would expect from taking such a hit, but I did suffer some spinal injuries that gave me problems with my hip, back, and knees. Needless to say, going to the gym was out of the question for me. Even though I was injured, I didn't give up. First I began physical therapy right away. And secondly, once I was able to move a little better, I began to think of ways that I could train at home. So if you can't afford to go a gym, I've got some great moves that will help you strengthen and tone your body right at home. Be aware that training at home takes a lot of motivation because there are so many distractions.

I know that because of cost and time that it's not always possible to make it to a gym. There are many exercise routines you can do at home. If you find yourself short on time, money, and/or find yourself stuck at home for whatever reason, you can still get a great workout right at home. Training at home takes a special kind of motivation. Get motivated by asking God in your prayers the night before to help motivate you to get up and do what you ought to do. Rebuke those demons of laziness the night before. Learning how to strength train at home is as simple as unitizing the things that are around you to create resistance for your muscles. The following is in no way an all inclusive list of the exercises you can perform at home. They are all birthed out my imagination, motivation, and desire to stay fit no matter what my circumstances are. To maintain our fitness, we must have a no excuses attitude, with severe sickness being the only exception.

For the upper body, you can:

- Use canned goods; perform bicep curls, tricep extension, and shoulder raises, and chest press, and a bent-over back press of alternating arm back row.

- Do pushups using the floor, the wall, a chair, or a stair step to work the chest and the triceps.

- Do tricep dips off of a chair.

- Do punches with cans.

For the midsection, do:

Abdominal

- Crunches on the floor (do for the middle, lower, and side)

- Lifting the knees to the chest in slow motion

- Lifting the knees to the chest from a sitting position

For the lower body, you can do:

- Calve raises on the stairs or on the box (a hard boxes with some books or other flat surfaced items inside)

- Work the quads, hams, and glutes by adding resistance to a regular squat. With your feet shoulder-width apart holding a can on each side of the body or placing a book bag on your back full of cans and then squatting.

- Note: To guarantee proper form, place a chair behind you, enough so that when you began to motion downward to perform, the upper part of your butt will slightly touch the edge of the seat. This way, you will know that you are going low enough to work the muscles.

Work the quads, inner thigh, and butt by adding resistance to a wide-stance squat (legs open wide in a standing position) by using a bottle of laundry detergent, extra-large can, or medium-size storage bin (used for food or clothes, that is half way or all the way filled).

Work the outer thigh by doing a repeated set of side leg lifts, by placing the hands on the hip and lifting the opposite leg. Add resistance to this by holding a can on the thigh of the leg being lifted.

Leg extensions can be performed by sitting in a kitchen chair, placing an ankle weight, or a small plastic bag with some cans (how many depends on your level of strength), tied with a knot on both ankles, and extending the legs forward. You can also strength train the legs at home by climbing stairs two or three steps at a time.

Calorie Buster Routines: These are fast pace movements

1. Calorie Buster:	Muscles Trained
15–25 jumping jacks	Heart/shoulders/legs
10–25 pushups hops (Knees bent)	Chest/triceps/back
Squat and to the side twist (15–25 to each side)	Quads/ hams/oblique
15–30 stomach bicycles (on the floor)	Upper/middle/lower abs

Jump rope for two minutes or 20–25 jumping jacks)
(Repeat three to five times

Beginners: start at ten and/or fifteen reps
Intermediate: start out at 20–25 reps
Advanced: do 25–30 reps

Modification: if you have knee problems and cannot jump, simply do the jumping jack motion without doing the actual jump.

Make It a Challenge

Jumping Jacks: use 5 or 10 pound weights or cans for jumping jacks and turn the upward arm motion into a shoulder press.

No weights, no problem Squat and side twist: hold a medicine ball or two canned items of equal weight.

Total workout: place cans or books in a book bag, place it on your back (adjust the strap so the bag is close to the body), and perform the entire routine.

Variation: first do the total routine at ten or fifteen reps, and then increase by two to five reps with each round of the routine. You can also do it in reverse.

Straight cardio: Run up one, two, or three flights of stairs; stop; do ten to twenty-five jumping jacks; run back down the stairs; and jump rope for three minutes. Repeat three to six times.

Strength training: in the gym

For the single muscle group, you can choose one, two, o three of any exercise to complete as part of you routine. You can do a total body workout or focus on lower body one day and upper body the next. It's totally up to you.

For legs, do twelve to twenty reps with 3, 5, 10-, 15-, or 20-pound dumbbells for three to four sets. You can also strap on a book bag, use cans, and/or add ankle weights to make the exercise more challenging.

Leg Extensions

1. Sitting: extending legs forward while sitting upright/back strait in a chair.

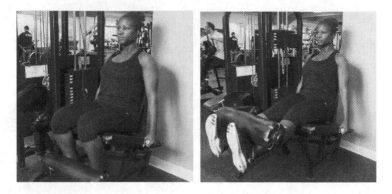

2. Standing: hands on the hips, raise leg up toward chest and extend out, bring leg down toward floor, tap the toes and repeat.

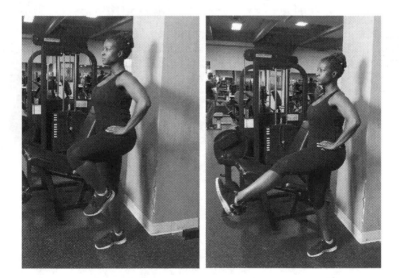

Variation: Keep the leg up and just continue to extend for twelve to twenty-five reps and then switch.

Lunges; Quads, Hams, Glutes,

1. Climb stairs two by two

2. Frontal Lunges

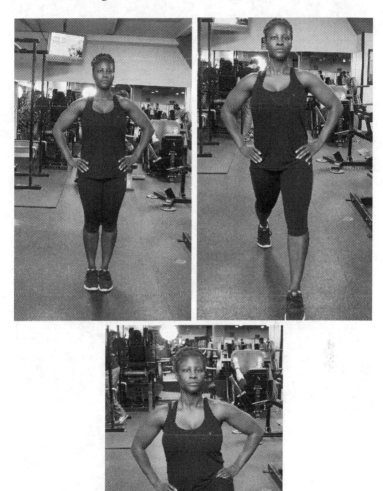

3. Side to Side Lunge Movement

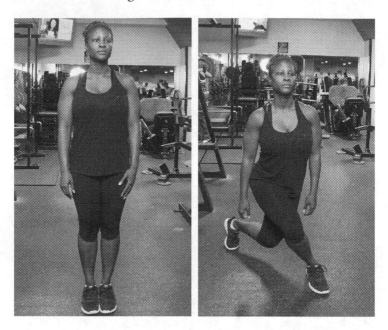

4. Posterior Lunges

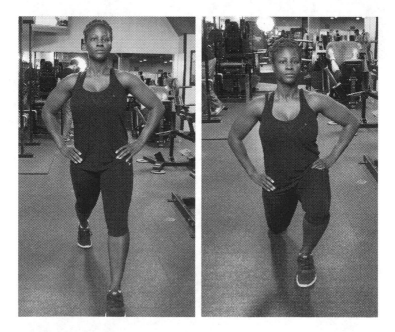

Squats: Quads, Hams, Butt, Inner Thigh

1. Bench Squat;

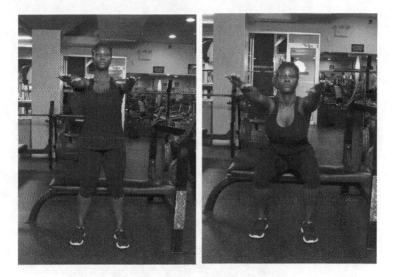

2. Pile squat (wide leg dip with weight in hand)

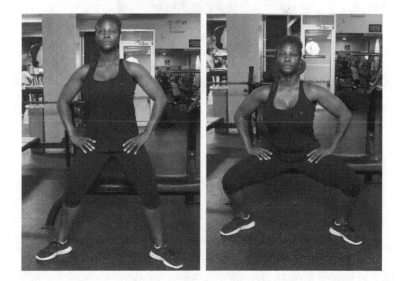

Heel raises: calves

1. Double legs

2. Single Leg

3. Both legs off the floor with dumbbells

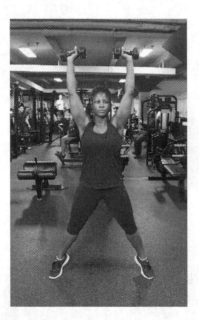

Lying back leg raise; abductors (inner thigh)

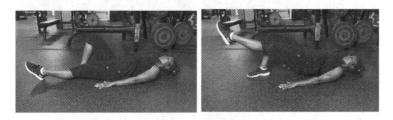

Lying or standing leg lifts; adductors (outer thigh)

*Both can be done using ankle weights or a heavy book

Posterior leg lifts; standing or on the floor (butt)
With or without weights

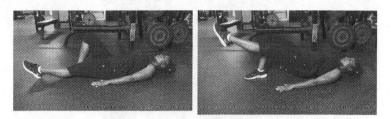

Upper body: can be done with cans, evenly filled bottles of liquid with handles, broomstick, and if available 5, 8, 10, 12, and 15 pound dumbbells. Do three to five sets of twelve to twenty reps.

Shoulders:
Shoulder press

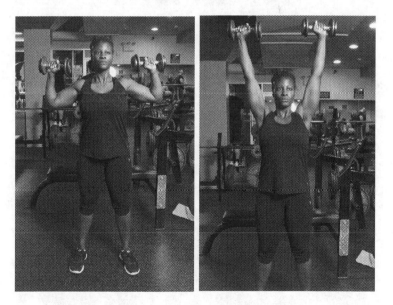

Lateral raises-
Frontal raises

Frontal /Lateral raise combo

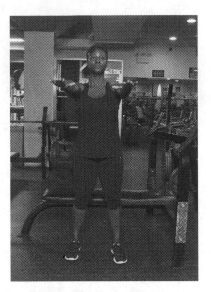

Back:
Standing/bent over lateral press

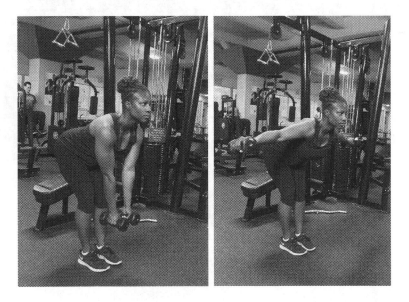

Bent single arm lateral press

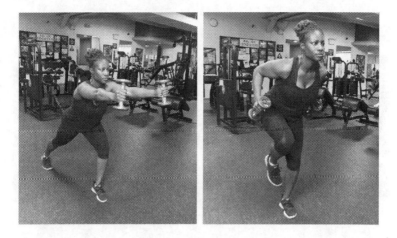

Pull-ups (broomstick or bar evenly positioned on two chairs.

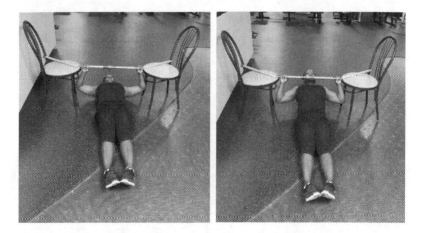

Chest:

1. Chest press; bent elbow or strait elbow (on the bench, floor or leaned back in a chair)

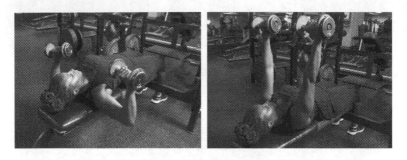

Pushups

2. Standing frontal press (strait elbows or bent elbows)

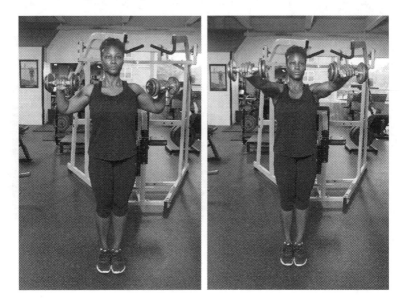

Biceps:

1. Bicep curls

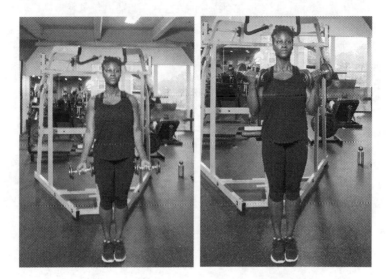

2. V- Curls

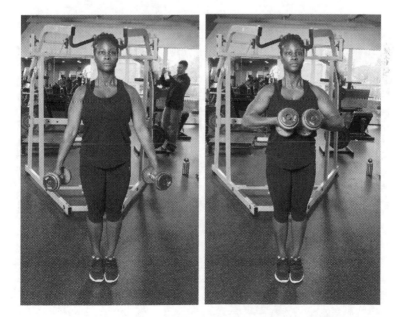

3. Lateral curls

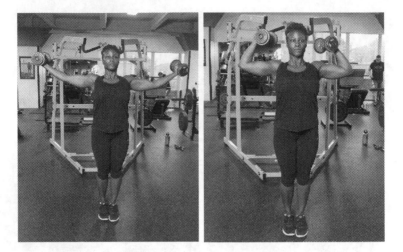

Triceps:

Triceps extension (standing or lying with arms over head, two arms or alternating) Bench dips

1. Level 1

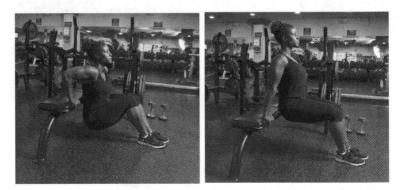

2. Level 2

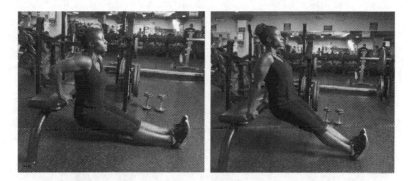

3. Level 3

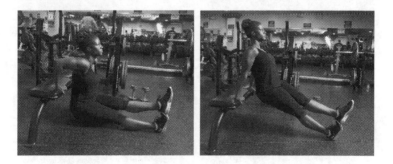

Abs: one to three exercises per section of abs, three or four sets each (again depending on the time you have.

Ten to twenty reps

Four second count up, hold for two seconds, then four second count down. Only do as many as you can handle without changing your posture. If posture begins to fall off, stop, rest for twenty to thirty seconds, and then begin a new set.

1. Basic Crunch

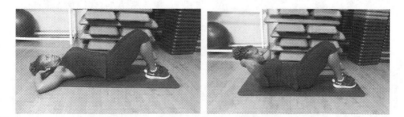

Safety Tip- to keep from pulling on the neck by find a dot on the ceiling and focus on it for the entire movement. This will keep the back, head and neck in the correct posture and alignment

2. Reverse crunch (lower and middle)

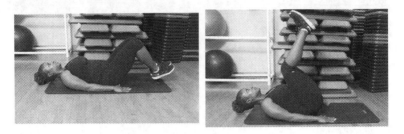

Safety Tip- If there are lower back issues tap the heels to the floor at the end of the movement to alleviate pressure off the back.

3. Oblique

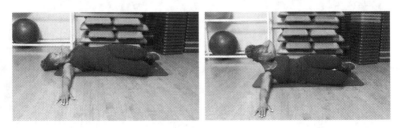

Safety Tip- follow the same tip as with crunches

4. Bicycle Crunch (total abdominal exercise; good when short on time)

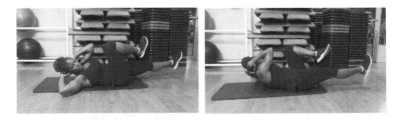

5. Crunch with clap

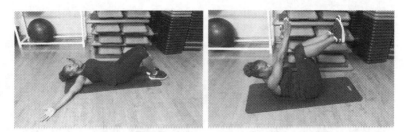

Two or More Muscle Groups

If you are short on time or want or simply want to dramatically increase calorie burn during strength training, here are some exercises you can do that work two or more muscle at the same time:

1. Squat and curl (add a shoulder press)

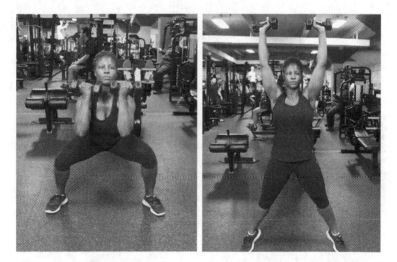

2. Squat and calve raise

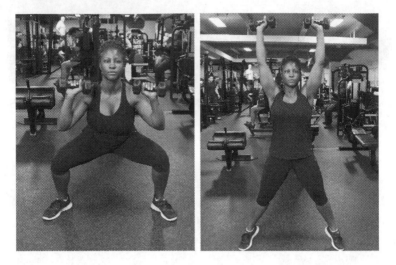

* If you feel any discomfort in the lower back, modify your squat by using a chair or bench, and simply sit and stand to mimic the squatting motion. Sitting down will take pressure off your lower back.

3. Lunge and curl (walking, or stationary; to the front, back or side)

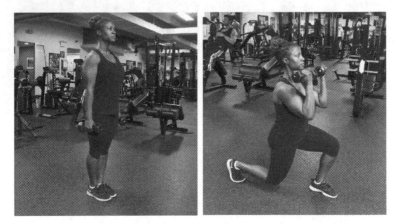

4. Lunge and overhead tricep extension.

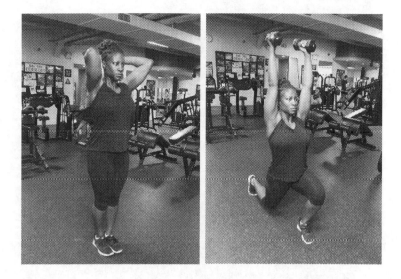

5. Dead lift and calve raise (You can also add a bicep curl.)

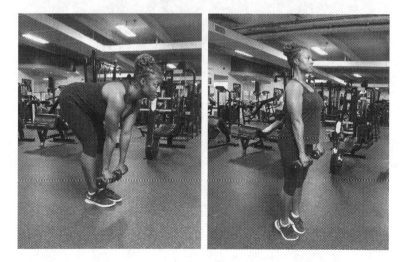

6. Back press and knee in

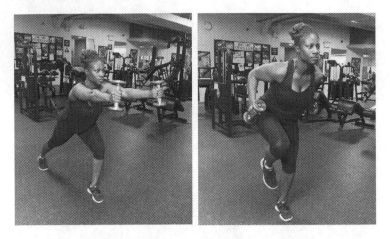

7. Triceps extension with knee in

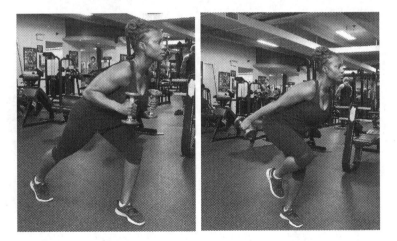

8. Butt bridge with overhead triceps exception

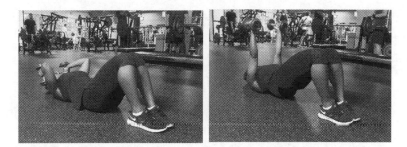

9. Butt bridge with chest press

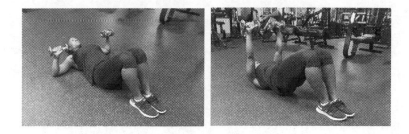

10. Lying chest press with reverse crunch

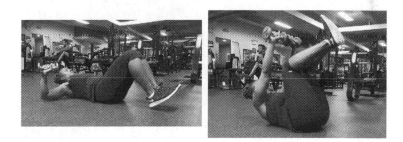

Making Strength Training Challenging

There are many ways to make your workout tougher without adding more weights.

On single muscle group or limb movement, adding a pulse motion to the move can really make it a lot more challenging. Pulsing is done by bringing the movement half the way through, returning to the start position, and then completing a full movement. You can do a one count pulse to start and graduate to doing a two to ten count pulse.

You can also do a set of pulses followed by a set of full extension. For example a ten-count shoulder press pulse set followed by a full extension press of ten reps, and then rest.

You can also perform a super set routine where you do two different exercises for the same muscle group back to back, only taking a rest at the completion of both exercises for thirty to sixty seconds. Two to four total sets is sufficient, unless you want to do more, and the muscle is not too fatigued. Remember, the most important thing is posture and form, not how many reps or sets you can do.

Combating Laziness

An at home workout can be just as effective as going to the gym, but in order to do so you must be motivated to get up and do it. There are times that I have had to trick myself so that I would get up. I set my alarm fifteen to ten minutes before I really have to get up; that way when I hit the snooze three times, I will still be getting up on time. Once I'm up, I go into the bathroom and pray for energy and motivation. I also have to talk directly to those demons of laziness and cancel their assignment against me, after which I ask God to give me focus and determination. Here are some other things you can do:

- Set aside a specific time the day before.

- Put on some upbeat spiritual music, or other feel good music

- Make a plan of what exercises you are going to do.

- If possible, don't take any calls before the time you are going to begin your routine.

- Have a healthy snack or small meal before you begin.

- If there are people around the home, who have a tendency to interrupt you, cordially and lovingly ask them to respect the time you have set aside to exercise, and if they give you problems about it, ask God to cause them to be understanding.

- Got kids no problem!!! Let them join in (its good bonding)

- Mommas… Strap that baby in the carrier on your back or chest and keep it movin! I did it- and lost 60 pounds of baby weight in 18 months (190 to 130 pounds)

In fact the photos for this chapter were taken only 10 months after giving birth!-Hence the all black! (LOL). I opted to show my real body doing real things and not a fitness model, because I thought it was important to illustrate that fitness is a process, a lifestyle, and choice. There will always be reasons not to exercise and stay fit, there will always be things happening, some good(having a baby), and some bad (having an injury) that can throw us off course, but when you really resolve to be healthy, and fit for the kingdom even during a set-back you are planning for your come back! The difference between those who succeed and fail at this is this: They both might not necessarily like the work that must be put in, but the successful group does it anyway- they subordinate how they feel to the overall goal at hand and the outcome they want to achieve.

Chapter 6

Reading Food Labels

The correction of discipline is the way to life.
(Proverbs 6:23)

Reading food labels can be pretty confusing. Understanding what constitutes a serving can be even more baffling. Because of this, most people ignore food nutritional labels. And very rarely do those who do read food labels eat only the suggested serving size. Because we have established that God cares about how we treat our bodies and what goes into them, we need to make an effort to understand food labels a little better.

The Bible tells us that discipline corrects us and is the way to life. Discipline takes focus, determination, and often times someone who God has place in our lives to be brutally honest with us and supply us with correct information. In this instance, being disciplined at paying attention to food labels and eating only what has been suggested by the label (or your nutritional professional), gives us the freedom necessary to enjoy a life of physical health. The enjoyment and freedom experienced comes from being disciplined enough to eat what you love without going overboard. Sticking to serving sizes/and or portions consistent with your fitness goals will free you from the guilt that most people experience when they consistently make the wrong food choices and/or eat too much.

For example, instead of having a pint of ice cream, you might have a half cup with some fruit and light whipped cream; you still to get to eat the ice cream (which is usually about 230 calories per half cup), but you have not eaten enough to blow all the hard work and start to condemn yourself. Self-condemnation as the result of guilt is one of the leading things that causes people to give up in this area of life. But remember:" there is no longer any condemnation for those of us who belong to Christ Jesus; For the Spirit has freed you" (Rom. 8:1–2). The following information on understanding food labels will give you the freedom to make better food choices and the freedom to enjoy the healthy lifestyle that God intends for all of us.

Terms and Definitions

Serving Sizes

The Food Guide Pyramid recommends a general dietary intake by food group in quantities called servings. Serving sizes were developed based on the amount of food typically consumed in one sitting, and the quantity of nutrients. These are the current general recommendations for what we should consume from each food group.

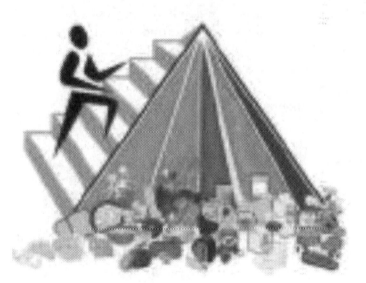

Courtesy www.grg.org

Each color of the food pyramid represents a food group. orange for grains, green for veggies, red for fruits, blue for milk, purple for meat and beans, and yellow for oils. These are the current general recommendations for what we should consume from each food group.

Bread, rice, pasta: 6–11 servings
Fruit: 2.5 cups (1 medium apple, banana, or orange, or 3/4 C. juice)

Vegetables: 2.5cups per day

Meat, poultry, fish, dry beans, eggs, and nuts: 5.5oz servings (2–3 oz. cooked meat: the size and height of a deck of cards, 1 egg, ½ C. cooked beans)

Milk, yogurt, and cheese: 2–3 servings, or 3 cups a day (1 C. milk or yogurt, 1 ½ oz. cheese: the length and thickness of your middle finger)

Fats, oils, sweets: use sparingly "Most Fats should come from, fish nuts and vegetable oil, limit solid fats such as butter, margarine, or lard". These servings represent what we should generally consume in one day. This is for general overall health. For specific advice for serving amounts for your specific fitness goal consulting with a fitness nutritionist can help you determine your more individualized needs.

Because of more current research and understanding in the area of nutrition, there is a new food pyramid being proposed, The New pyramid emphasizes daily exercise and weight control, it places whole grains such as brown rice, whole grain whole wheat pastas and breads at the bottom of the pyramid (meaning we should eat more), and places white starches, like white bread, pasta and potatoes at the top of the pyramid along with sweets (meaning we should eat these the least)

New perspectives on health and nutrition acknowledges the many dangers of consuming too much of the so called "white starches" and high glycemic carbohydrates (discussed in Chapter 8).

For people trying to lose weight and tone up, overconsumption of white starches can be counterproductive. One of the main reasons is that the so-called white starches turn to sugar in the body so quick, that the body does not have time to fully register the volume of food that has been consumed. The result is people tend to overeat white starches, because they have to eat more of a white starch (versus a whole grain or brown starch) in order to feel full.

The Science

Overeating, particularly when consuming white starches, causes an overproduction of insulin (the hormone that assists in the storage of fat). In other words, the body experiences a sugar high after eating white starches. After the high, there is a crash (the feeling of sleepiness), which causes the body to crave something else that will give it the same experience. Although the body is craving the food, it does not mean the body really needs the calories. So what happens is that our craving manifests itself into overeating. On the other hand, whole grain starches cause insulin levels to rise more slowly, giving the body the feeling of satisfaction sooner and making us feel full longer, which tends to cause most people to eat less. I will explain this process in more detail in Chapter 8.

Eating a larger quantity of green veggies with meals along with a lean meat, one whole grain starch, in addition to using primarily plant oils (such as extra virgin olive oil, safflower oil, and grape seed oil) as the source of fat when we cook can help increase the feeling of satiety (feeling full), when eating.

Discrepancies between the Current Food Pyramid and Food Labels

Serving sizes on food labels do not necessarily match the Food Guide Pyramid. For example, the pyramid considers a ½ cup of rice as a serving. Most food labels list the serving size as 1cup. So according to the food pyramid, 1 cup of rice equals 2 servings of rice. In general, a cup is ok, any differences depend the individual nutritional needs of the person.

Serving size does not necessarily correspond with package size. For example, as we discussed in the last chapter when we talked about portion control, a bottled beverage may define 1 serving as 8 fluid ounces, while the bottle contains 20 ounces. Drinking the entire bottle would be the equivalent of consuming 2½ servings of the beverage.

Food Labels

Food labels express serving sizes in household measures (tablespoons), and metric measures (ounces and grams). They list contents by weight and measure. Ingredients are listed from most to least. Whatever the product contains the most of will be listed first, whatever it contains the least will be listed last. Most packaged foods are required to display a Standard Label of Nutritional Information.

Nutrition Facts Panel

1. States the Serving size and serving per container.

2. Calories per serving and calories from fat.

3. Nutrient amounts and percentages of Daily Values, which include:

   a. Total fat (lipid)

   b. Cholesterol

   c. Sodium

   d. Total carbohydrate, with the break down showing dietary fiber and sugars

   e. Protein

   f. Vitamin A, Vitamin C, calcium, and iron, expressed as percentages of Daily Values. Daily values are based on the government recommended amount of each nutrient it believes is necessary for the optimal health of an individual. For men, the percentage of each nutrient consumed each day is based on a 2,500 caloric intake, and for women a 2,000 calorie a day intake. Generally men need more than women to maintain optimal health. Below is an example of a food label.

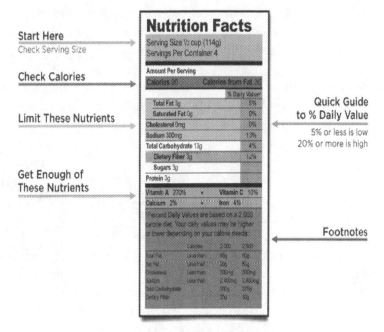

Start Here
Check Serving Size

Check Calories

Limit These Nutrients

**Get Enough of
These Nutrients**

Nutrition Facts

**Quick Guide
to % Daily Value**
5% or less is low
20% or more is high

Footnotes

CALORIES PER GRAM : FAT 9 CARBOHYDRATES 4 PROTIEN 4

The total number of calories in a given food reflects the grams of carbohydrate, lipid (fat), and protein.

1 gram of carbohydrates = 4 calories
1 gram of protein = 4 calories
1 gram of fat = 9 calories

In the above nutrition label, the total number of calories for 1 serving is 90. There are 3 grams of fat, 13 grams of carbohydrates, and 3 grams of protein. To figure out how many calories you are getting from each nutrient in this food, you would simply multiply the amount of listed grams of each by the amount of calories found in one gram of each.

For example:

Carbohydrates: 13g x 4 calories = 52 calories
Protein: 3g x 4 calories = 12 calories
Fat: 3g x 9 calories = 27 calories

Total = 91, the extra 1 calorie possibly being a miscalculation by the food labeler but the point is to know how the calories in your foods add up and where they come from.

Notice that in this can of food there are 4 servings, so consuming the entire contents would quadruple the amount of calories from fat carbohydrates and protein being consumed.

Here the majority of the calories are coming from carbohydrates. Depending on the grams of each nutrient in any given food, an item with the same amount of calories could also have a higher percentage of calories that come from fat or protein.

This explains why two food products with the same amount of calories (when eaten in excess) have different effects on the body in terms of weight gain, loss, or maintenance, especially where a large amount of the total calories are coming from fat. Think about the difference between the 100 calorie cookie (and we all eat more than one) and 100 calories of broccoli.

Now that we have cleared the air on that, let's take a look at some other things we commonly see advertised on food labels, such as fat-free, sugar-free, low carb, high protein, and net carbs.

- *Reduced fat* means that a product has 25 percent less fat than the regular version of the product.

- *Light* means that the product has 50 percent less fat than the regular product.

- *Low-fat* means a product has less than 3 grams of fat per serving.

- *Fat-free* means that there is no fat in the product, but beware, this is not always what it's cracked up to be; things low in fat are usually so high in sugar you may be better off buying the regular product

- *Low carb* products are usually high fat.

- *High protein*: is not always better because many of these products leave you feeling hungry and tired because of the lack of enough carbohydrates, which is the body's chief source of energy.

- *Sugar-free* does not always mean low-calorie.

Ingredients

Much of the food we consume is made up of all kinds of ingredients; some that are naturally occurring and others that are added in. Substances that are added to food are called food additives.

Food Additives

High Fructose Corn Syrup (HFCS) is only one of many, and most common things added to the foods we consume to make them what they are. These substances called *food additives*[28] "are substances or a mixture of substances other than the basic foodstuff which is present in food as a result of any phase production, processing, packaging, and storage of food."[29]

Nutritional additives are used to add vitamins and minerals to foods that may have been stripped during the production process and/or to improve nutritional value. Without them, milk would lack the adequate amount of vitamin D. *Cosmetic additives* "enhance" the smell, taste, and look of food. Without them, strawberry ice cream would not be pink. *Preservatives* are additives that help keep food fresh. Without them, food would spoil much quicker. *Processing additives* aid in the process of preparing, storing, and shipping food. Some of these particular items become a part of the food content by virtue of being packaged and stored in a particular manner. Without these in foods, it would be more difficult to make, store, package, and ship them. It would probably make many products much more expensive as well.

---

[28] Patricia Redline, and Diane Nelson, *Food Additives: What Are They?* (Iowa University, National Central Regional Publication, 1993), pg438.

[29] Ibid

While many people believe that additives are potentially harmful and unnecessary, in societies where few people produce their own food such as the United States, food additives make it possible for consumers to enjoy food that is "flavorful, nutritious, convenient, readily available, safe, abundant, varied, and reasonably priced."[30]

What scares people the most about additives is their big long names found within the ingredients list. A common one is *monoglyceride* or *lecithin*. These are additives that are used during the process of making products such as salad dressing and pudding.

Whether we eat out or in and/or buy products that are premade or make food from scratch at home, all foods are made of chemical compounds that determine the way food smells, looks, tastes, and the type of nutrients it contains.

The chart below illustrates in more detail each class of additives, their names (found in the list of food ingredients on the nutrition label) and their uses:

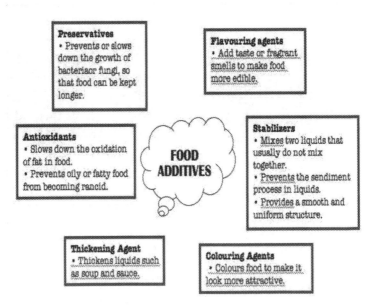

---

[30] Ibid

Top 10 Food Additives to Avoid

Additive	Known as	Used in	Reasons to avoid
Aspartame	E951	So-called "diet" or "sugar free" products (including diet coke, coke zero), jello, desserts, sugar free gum, drink mixes, table top sweeteners, cereal, breath-mints, puddings, kool-aid, ice tea, chewable vitamins, toothpaste, cough syrup	Aspartame is not your friend. Aspartame is a neurotoxin and carcinogen. Known to erode intelligence and affect short-term memory, the components of this toxic sweetener may lead to a wide variety of ailments including brain tumor, diseases like lymphoma, diabetes, multiple sclerosis, Parkinson's, Alzheimer's, fibromyalgia, chronic fatigue, depression and anxiety attacks, dizziness, headaches, nausea, mental confusion and seizures.
High Fructose Corn Syrup	HFCS	most processed foods, breads, candy, flavored yogurts, salad dressings, canned vegetables, cereals	High fructose corn syrup (HFCS) is a highly-refined artificial sweetener which has become the number one source of calories in America. HFCS packs on the pounds faster than any other ingredient, increases your LDL ("bad") cholesterol levels, and contributes to the development of obesity and diabetes.
Monosodium Glutamate	MSG / E621	Chinese food, potato chips, many snacks, chips, cookies, seasonings, most Campbell Soup products, frozen dinners, lunch meats	MSG is used as a flavor enhancer but also effects the neurological pathways of the brain and disengages the "I'm full" function which results, for many, in weight gain. MSG is an excito-toxin, and regular consumption may result in depression, disorientation, eye damage, fatigue, headaches, and obesity.
Trans Fat	Partially hydrogenated vegetable oils	margarine, chips and crackers, baked goods, fast foods	Trans fat increases LDL cholesterol levels while decreasing HDL ("good") cholesterol, increases the risk of heart attacks, heart disease and strokes, and contributes to increased inflammation, diabetes and other health problems.
Food Dyes Blue #1 & Blue #2 Red #3 & Red #40 Yellow #6 & Yellow Tartrazine	E133 E124 E110 E102	fruit cocktail, maraschino cherries, cherry pie mix, ice cream, candy, bakery products, American cheese, macaroni and cheese	Artificial colorings, may contribute to behavioral problems like ADD and ADHD in children and lead to a significant reduction in IQ. Animal studies have linked other food colorings to cancer.
Sodium Sulphite	E221	wine and dried fruit	According to the FDA, approximately one in 100 people are sensitive to sulphites in food. Individuals who are sulfite sensitive may experience asthma, headaches, breathing problems and rashes.
Sodium Nitrate/Sodium Nitrite	E250	hotdogs, bacon, ham, luncheon meat, cured meats, corned beef, smoked fish or any other type of processed meat	Sodium Nitrate is the chemical that turns meats bright red but it's highly carcinogenic once it enters the human digestive system. There, it forms a variety of nitrosamine compounds that enter the bloodstream and wreak havoc with a number of internal organs; the liver and pancreas in particular. This toxic chemical is linked to many cancers.
BHA and BHT	E320	used as a preservative in potato chips, gum, cereal, frozen sausages, enriched rice, lard, shortening, candy, jello	This common preservative keeps foods from changing color, changing flavor or becoming rancid. Effects the neurological system of the brain, alters behavior and has potential to cause cancer. BHA and BHT are oxidants which form cancer-causing reactive compounds in your body.
Sulphur Dioxide	E220	used as a preservative in beers, soft drinks, dried fruit, juices, cordials, wine, vinegar, and potato products	Sulphur additives are toxic. Adverse reactions include; bronchial problems, asthma, hypotension, flushing tingling sensations or anaphylactic shock. It destroys vitamins B1 and E in the body. Not recommended for consumption by children.
Potassium Bromate	E924	used to increase volume in bread and bread-rolls	Potassium bromate is known to cause cancer in animals. Even small amounts in bread can create problems for humans.

(Courtesy foodmatters.tv)

In the United States, the use of food additives is regulated by the Food and Drug Administration (FDA).[31] They regulate the type of food an additive can be used in and how much. However, manufacturers, not the FDA, are responsible for proving that the additive is safe. "Safety has not been defined by the law but has been interpreted by the FDA to be *a reasonable certainly of no harm under intended use conditions.*"[32]. The use of additives is continually reviewed and "modified or withdrawn as necessary" by the FDA, they are never permanently approved.

---

[31] Ibid

[32] Ibid

Sulfites

Sulfites are used for a number of "food technological functions" (i.e., the making of food products). Sulfites are most used in dried fruits and vegetables, wines, vinegar, instant potatoes and meats, and are used to preserve taste and color of foods. In a list of ingredients, sulfites are identified as sulfur dioxide, sodium metabisufite, sodium bisulfite, potassium metabisulfite, and potassium bisulfite.

For many, sulfites have caused adverse affects. If you think that there are ingredients in your food that have an adverse affect on you, it is best to take the time to research the ingredients and/or limit the amount of the product you consume, if you can narrow it down to a specific product.

High-Fructose Corn Syrup and Wheat Gluten

High-fructose corn syrup and wheat gluten (an elastic protein substance that gives cohesiveness to dough)[33], are two food additives that can have an adverse affect on the ability to lose and/or gain weight, even with a healthy eating plan. Their uses are so widespread that they are hard to avoid, unless you are willing to switch over to products that are a little more expensive but use other types of additives that serve the same purpose but have little or no underlying affect on your waistline.

High-Fructose Corn Syrup:

It is believed that there are certain ingredients in our everyday foods that may be "culpable" for society's expanding waistline and the inability to lose those extra inches.[34] One such ingredient is high-fructose corn syrup (HFCS), which is the newer form of corn syrup.

HFCS is a form of sugar derived from corn syrup, and it is most commonly used to sweeten everyday foods. Corn syrup, also known as glucose syrup, is made from corn starch. In its liquid form, it is used to keep foods moist and to keep them from spoiling too soon.

---

[33] LaZelle Blue Brady, *Weight Gain, Cravings, and Genetics* www.epicinternet.com/aricles/article-037274.htm.

[34] www.supermarketguru.com/page.cfm/2925 "Why Critics Say HFCS Is the Four Letter Word ... That Goes Right to Our Waistlines. September 20, 2003.

HFCS contains a high level of fructose, the same type of sugar found in fruits. Because it is 75 percent sweeter than regular sugar, is cheaper, and mixes well with many foods, manufacturers began using it as a primary sweetener for foods in the 1970s. HFCS is used in a variety of products including canned goods, baking and ice cream products, juices, jellies, candies, cookies, syrups, yogurt, ketchup, breakfast cereals, pasta sauces, jams, jellies, and especially sodas.

It is believed HFCS causes weight gain because it seems to have the affect of stimulating the appetite rather than reducing it and because the fructose converts to fat more than any other sugar[35]. While the corn syrup, aka glucose, in HFCS is used by the body as an immediate source of energy, the fructose is not digested as easily by the body and is converted into fat.

When glucose is digested, it stimulates an insulin response, which in turn stimulates the production of the hormone leptin, the hormone that sends the message to the brain that prompts us to stop eating.

When fructose is ingested, it does not stimulate the production of insulin, and without this, the hormone that prompts us to stop eating isn't stimulated either. HFCS may therefore contribute to increased food intake and weight gain.

So What Do You Do?

First, if you want to start losing some serious weight, stop drinking soda and processed fruit juices, which have about 8 teaspoons of HFCS per serving. Try to choose products that list the ingredient toward the bottom of the list. Ingredients are listed in order of how much of it is present in the food.

Wheat Gluten

Wheat Gluten is an ingredient most commonly found in breads. It gives cohesiveness to the breads. Many people are allergic to wheat gluten

---

[35] /www.mercola.com/2004/apr/10/corn/_fat.htm "Six Reasons Why Corn Is Making You Fat."

and don't even know it. An allergy to wheat gluten involves the inability of the body to digest the substance. The undigested wheat gluten forms into a "sticky acidic protein paste."[36] This paste lines the small intestines, causing a blockage of the "nutrient receptors." This means other nutrients from the foods being consumed are not being absorbed into the blood stream, leaving the body starving and craving more food. In other words, you have eaten, but because the body is not getting the nutrients from the food, the body sends out a signal (a food craving), which can cause overconsumption. Unabsorbed food causes bloating because the digested food just sits in the small intestines. When trying to lose weight, the blockage of the nutrient receptors makes it hard for the food that is digested to be absorbed enough to cause a change in weight. The best way to determine if this ingredient is the root of your dietary dilemma is to switch to bread made without wheat gluten, such as products made with *brown rice and/or quinoa* for a month or two. If you feel less bloated, and/or if it is your goal to, begin to lose weight, then this is a pretty good indication that a food allergy to gluten does exist. You can also ask your doctor to perform a blood test for celiac disease; this can tell you if you just have a gluten sensitivity or a more serious issue like celiac disease.

Artificial Sweeteners[37]

Artificial sweeteners are used as low-calorie alternatives to sugar and are used to make low-calorie food products. They include aspartame, saccharin, and sucralose.

Aspartame is a low-calorie sweetener with a sugar like taste that is approximately 200 times sweeter than sucrose. Aspartame is unique among low-calorie sweeteners in that it is completely broken down by the body to its components—the amino acids, aspartic acid, and phenylalanine, and a small amount of methanol. These components are found in much greater amounts in common foods, such as meat, milk, fruits, and vegetables, and are used in the body in the same ways whether they come from aspartame or common foods. Aspartame is one of the most thoroughly studied food ingredients ever. In 1981, aspartame

---

[36] Ibid., 2.
[37] www.caloriecontrol.org.
www.pccnaturalmarkets.com/health/Food_Guide/Natural_Sweeteners.htm.

was approved for use in tabletop sweeteners and various foods and dry beverage mixes, making it the first low-calorie sweetener approved by the U.S. Food and Drug Administration (FDA) in more than twenty-five years. In 1983, the FDA approved aspartame for use in carbonated beverages followed by a number of other product category approvals over the next thirteen years, leading to a general use approval in foods and beverages in 1996.

Today, aspartame has established itself as an important component in the taste of thousands of foods and beverages without all the calories of sugar. Currently, aspartame is found in more than 6,000 products and is consumed by over 200 million people around the world.

Saccharin has been used to sweeten foods and beverages without calories or carbohydrates for over a century. Its use was considerable during the sugar shortages of the two world wars, particularly in Europe. For many people, saccharin is an integral part of their lifestyle. It is particularly important to those whose diets require a restriction of caloric or carbohydrate intake, such as persons with diabetes. Most health practitioners favor the use of a non-caloric sweetener like saccharin in weight reduction and for people with diabetes. Saccharin continues to be important for a wide range of low-calorie and sugar-free food and beverage applications. It is used in such products as soft drinks, tabletop sweeteners, baked goods, jams, chewing gum, canned fruit, candy, dessert toppings, and salad dressings. Saccharin also is used in cosmetic products, vitamins, and pharmaceuticals. The current availability of saccharin and other low-calorie sweeteners, such as aspartame, acesulfame potassium, cyclamate, and sucralose, allows manufacturers to utilize a "multiple sweetener approach"—using the most appropriate sweetener, or combination of sweeteners, for a given product. No low-calorie sweetener is perfect for all uses. However, a variety of sweeteners enables the development of a much wider range of new, good-tasting, low-calorie products to meet consumer demand. Also, a variety of low-calorie sweeteners provides products with increased stability, improved taste, lower production costs and more choices for the consumer.

Sucralose is the only noncaloric sweetener made from sugar. Sucralose is derived from sugar and is 600 times sweeter than sucrose and tastes like sugar. It was first discovered in 1976, and was granted approval by the FDA on April 1, 1998, and approved for use in fifteen food and beverage categories. In 1999, it was approved as a "general purpose" sweetener. Sucralose has also been approved for use in foods and beverages in more than forty countries including Canada, Australia, and Mexico. Sucrolose is not utilized for energy in the body because it is not broken down like sucrose. It passes rapidly through the body virtually unchanged. Extensive tests over the past twenty years suggest that sucralose is safe and can be used by all populations, including pregnant women, nursing mothers, and children of all ages. Sucralose is said to be beneficial for individuals with diabetes because it has no effect on carbohydrate metabolism, short- or long-term blood glucose control, or insulin secretion. Sucralose is available as an ingredient for use in a broad range of foods and beverages under the name SPLENDA Brand Sweetener.

It has been cited that there are many side effects that can occurs from using sugar substitutes.[38] Side effects can be minor to severe. The longer the person consumes it, the more it increases the risks. Headaches/migraines, dizziness, nausea, weight gain, muscle spasms, depression, fatigue, insomnia, heart palpitations, vision and hearing problems, anxiety attacks, vertigo, memory loss, joint pain, emotional disorders, multiple sclerosis, lupus, chronic fatigue syndrome, brain tumors, brain cancer, diabetes, Parkinson's disease, Alzheimer's disease, epilepsy, birth defects, and mental retardation. These side effects have been seen the most with the long-term use of aspartame

Sucralose is an artificial sweetener made from sugar; it is a chlorinated sucrose derivative. Though considered "safer" than aspartame or saccharin by many, it is thought that there have not been enough *long-term* studies done on this product, and many believe it may be just as hazardous as some of its competitors.

Research in animal testing has shown the following side effects: chest pains, irritability, confusion, fatigue, shrunken thymus gland, enlarged liver and kidneys, reduced growth rate, decreased red blood cell count, hyperplasia of pelvis, miscarriage, decreased fetal body weights, changes

---

[38] www.pccnaturalmarkets.com/health/Food_Guide/Natural_Sweeteners.htm.

in mood, and diarrhea. There are *no long-term* studies on the effects of sucralose consumption.

Natural Sweeteners[39]

The different type of natural sweeteners that you might find within foods are: barley malt, brown rice syrup, concentrated fruit sweetener, date sugar, fructose, fruit juice concentrate, fruit juice sweeteners, Fruit Source®, glucose, honey, maple syrup, Stevia, and Sucanet®. These are usually found in all natural products in health food stores.

Stevia

Stevia is derived from a South American shrub *(Stevia rebaudiana)*. A good quality leaf is estimated to be 300 times sweeter than cane sugar, or sucrose. Also known as "honey leaf" and yerba dulce, stevia is not absorbed through the digestive tract, and is therefore non-caloric. Although Stevia adds sweetness to foods, it cannot be sold as a sweetener because the FDA considers it an unapproved food additive. However, under the provisions of the Dietary Supplement Health and Education Act (DSHEA) passed in 1994, Stevia can be sold as a dietary supplement. Stevia can be used as an alternative to products such as Equal and Splenda.

Change Today

- Get into the habit of reading food labels.

- Eat food according the food label, if you want to have your favorite ice cream, go ahead, but eat only the serving size. Add some fruit to it and non-fat whipped cream to replace the extra amount you're use to.

- Begin to document what you ate and how much of the food item you ate. For example, instead of writing "a bowl of cereal," write 1 cup (8 oz.) of cereal with 1 cup (8 oz.) of milk. Just keep a small notepad in your bag or in your pocket. I suggest you do it every

---

[39] www.pccnaturalmarkets.com/health/Food_Guide/Natural_Sweeteners.htm.

time you eat or drink something, because it will make you more aware, but if you forget, do it before you go to bed at night. But try to remember to do it right away, because most people might remember their meals, but most won't remember the handfull of M&Ms they had at two o'clock or the can of soda at five.

Prayer:

Father in the name of Jesus I thank you for the information
You provided. Let it get down into my spirit, and be brought to
My remembrance the next time I go food shopping, cook
A meal, and sit down to eat. Help me to be disciplined and
More cautious of what I put in my body, for it was beautifully
And wonderfully made by you and I appreciate it. To you be all the
Glory and honor for my body, the work of your hand. In Jesus name
Amen.

Chapter 7

Flex to Do Your Best

"I will instruct you and show you way to go;
with eye on you, I will give you counsel"
(Proverbs 32:8)

There are many stories illustrated in the Bible that talk about how rigid the scribes and Pharisees were. Jesus often referred to them as having hardened hearts. Because their hearts were hard, they lacked the love and mercy that was necessary to use the law as a way to build up the people they were leading and not break them down. When Jesus showed this type of love by healing people and forgiving their sins, he was often accused of breaking the law or violating some other social/cultural rules. In one such incidence, he was accused of working on the Sabbath because he healed a man's hand (Luke 3:1–6). So Jesus asked them, "Is it wrong to do good works on the Sabbath?" You see the Pharisees were strong in what they knew, but the hardness of hearts (lacking love and mercy), prevented them from really moving in the power of God through the law as Jesus did; they were spiritually inflexible. This spiritual inflexibility limited their effectiveness as leaders of God's people and caused them to reject the messiah and "the power that could make them godly" (2 Tim. 3:5).

Comparatively, when there are certain muscles in the body that are very tight (due to overuses and/or micro injuries), they are less flexible, making it difficult to perform certain exercises and/or get the full benefit out of the movement because of an inability to maintain the proper form associated with the exercise. In the same way the Pharisees overlooked the importance of love and mercy in their duties to teach and fulfill the law, most people overlook the importance of stretching, which helps restore muscles to a length that allows for better body movement.

It is important to work on flexibility as a normal part of your workout regimen. Being flexible allows the muscles to move as they should during strength training and cardiovascular exercises. "Poor flexibility leads to the development of *relative flexibility*,"[40] a condition where the body alters its movement pattern by recruiting other muscles not primary to the movement as the primary muscle so that you can complete the movement. Tight muscles are caused by muscles that are have become overactive because they are having to do all the work for other weaker muscles that surround it and/or micro injuries that happen overtime causing the muscles fiber to bunch up into knots. The knots are the little repairs that the body has made to the muscle. Over time, this bunching up of the muscle fibers causes the muscle to shorten. The best way to imagine this process is to think about a very long shoestring that has been tied in many knots. Eventually, the sting becomes very short. If you wanted to use it in your sneakers, it would no longer be long enough to do so. Tight muscles prevent flexibility because the muscle becomes too short (tight) to move as well as it should. For example, during squats, the primary movers are the quadriceps muscles located in the front part of the leg. But if the quadriceps are weak or inhibited because they are not flexible enough (tight and in a shortened state), the body places the load of performing the movement on other surrounding muscles, resulting in an improper movement pattern. To understand what I mean, try the following.

Stand up and raise your arms fully extended over your head. Then do a squat five times. Notice if your knees turn inward or outward. The turning of your knees is a demonstration of an altered movement developed by your body due to a lack of flexibility. The result of some tight, overworked muscles (which need to be stretched) compensating for weak lazy muscles (which need to be strengthened). Thus flexibility and strength training go hand and hand. Lack of flexibility and weak muscles, lead to muscle imbalances, making it difficult to maintain proper form and posture during strength training.

Improving Flexibility

Improving flexibility requires stretching tight muscles. This should typically be done before and after a workout. There are three levels of

---

[40] A. Clark and Rodney J. Corn, *NASM Optimum Performance Training for Fitness Professional* (National Academy of Sports Medicine, Calabasas, CA, 2001)

flexibility: corrective, active, and dynamic, which correspond to three levels of stretching: static, active, and dynamic.

Static stretching involves holding a stretch pose for twenty seconds or more. Holding the muscle for a prolonged period of time allows the soft tissue of the muscle to be relaxed (lengthening the muscle), which can help make movement easier. Static stretching can be used both before and after a workout. Pre-workout static stretching is typically for those who have postural distortions, as a form of corrective flexibility to help correct muscle imbalances, and can be typically used by all as part of a post-workout cool-down to bring the heart rate back down to it normal status. Static stretching should be done anywhere from four to eight weeks before moving on to the next level of flexibility, which involves active stretching, but can be longer depending on how bad the muscles imbalances are.

In addition to static stretches, it is also good to use a method called self-myofascial release[41] to loosen up the adhesions, also known as "knots" in the muscles. As explained earlier, tight muscles are the result of micro injuries that when repaired cause the muscle to knot up, and shorten, in the same way a shoestring as you tie knots in it becomes shorter and shorter. "Applying gentle force to the adhesion or knot" allows the muscle fibers to be "manipulated from a bundle position (that causes the adhesion), into an alignment that is straighter with the direction of the muscle."[42] In other words, it unties the knots that make the muscle tight, lengthening them again so that you have a better range of motion. "This process will help restore the body back to the optimal level of function."[43]

Self-myofacial release is done using a foam roller or a stick. The foam roller or stick is used to apply gentle force to tender areas of the muscle (which identify spots of adhesions). This is done by rolling the form or stick underneath a muscle area and slowly moving backward or forward in order to find tender areas. Once identified, the foam roller or stick is held in that place for thirty seconds "or until the discomfort is reduced by at least 75 percent."[44] Foam rollers can be found in most sporting good

[41] Ibid pg155
[42] Ibid pg 157.
[43] Ibid pg 157
[44] Ibid pg 157

stores of can be ordered online. Depending on the length, a foam roller will cost anywhere from five to twenty dollars. The 16-inch rollers are the most popular because they are longer and easier for most people to use.

It is suggested that self-myofacial release is done before static stretching, and it can be used as a cool-down after a workout. Active stretching is stretching that involves movement. Stretches are quicker and are only held in the stretch position for two to four seconds. The movement is typically repeated for five to ten repetitions, and this is used if no postural distortion movement patterns exist or they have been significantly reduced"[45] through static stretching and self-myofacial release. Active stretching is typically done for four to eight weeks before moving on to the next level of flexibility, which involves dynamic stretching.

Because there is more movement of the body involved in active stretching, it is better than static stretching for warming up the body before a workout, because it allows more blood flow and oxygen to be delivered to the muscles, making them better prepared to handle the demand of exercise activities performed during the workout.

Dynamic stretching involves the use of the body's momentum (force production) to stretch the muscles. The movement of these stretches typically mimic the types of movements that will be done during strength training, are continuous, and involve no to very little holding. An example of this is doing a set of walking lunges.

Dynamic stretches are typically performed as a pre-workout warm-up because the movements help to elevate the heart rate and increase blood and oxygen flow to the joints and muscles, making the body better prepared for the workout activity. Again, this form of stretching is only suggested if no postural distortion patterns exist or have been reduced.

---

[45] 45.Ibid Pg145

Putting It All Together

Your workout should therefore consist of:

A general warm up (five to ten minutes)

1. Self-myofacial release (for all)

2. Flexibility: static (for those with muscles imbalances and severe postural distortion), active or dynamic stretching (for those with more advanced levels of flexibility)

The workout activity

1. Cardio (two to five minute warm-up pace to start)

or

2. Weight training routine

A Cool-down (five to ten minutes, depending on how intense the workout activity was)

1. Slowing down the pace in the final two to three minutes of the cardio activity

and/or

2. Static stretching (for all)

It is very important not to ignore incorporating flexibility exercises into your routine. Now that you have a better understanding of why flexibility is important to reaching your fitness goals, do them every time you work out. In the same way that building up our relationship with God and serving him requires the integration of many different components, like prayer, study, fellowship, self-growth, creating a healthy and fit body requires that flexibility be one of the primary components, in order to produce the most optimal results.

Chapter 8

Understand What You Eat and Drink Carbohydrates, Protein, Fats, Fiber, and Water

As for Phillip, an angel of the Lord said to him, "Go south down the desert road that runs from Jerusalem to Gaza." So he started out, and met a treasure of Ethiopia, a eunuch of a great authority under Kandake the queen of Ethiopia. The eunuch had gone to Jerusalem to worship, and he was now returning. Seated in his carriage, he was reading aloud from the book of the prophet Isaiah. The Holy Spirit said to Phillip, "Go over and walk alongside the carriage." Phillip ran over and heard the man reading from the prophet Isaiah. Phillip asked, "Do you understand what you are reading?" The man replied, "How can I, unless someone instructs me?"
—Acts 8:26–31

In the above story taken from the book of Acts, we see a man who is reading the word of God, but has no understanding of what it is he is reading or the significance of what's being said. In the same fashion most of us eat, because we know how, and know we need to, but are unable to really give thoughtful consideration about what it is we are actually putting in our bodies, due in part to a lack of knowledge on the matter. Phillip asked the man if he understood what he was reading. And I ask you, do you understand what you're eating? As the story goes on, Phillip explains the scriptures to the eunuch. As a result, the man believes the good news- that Jesus the son of God, came to earth died for our sins, and because of the sacrifice he made , we have right standing with God if we choose to accept it, and then he gets baptized. Similarly, I believe that gaining a solid understanding of the food we eat can help us make decisions that will change the course of our heath, paralleling how the word of God through the book of Isaiah and the help of Philip caused the eunuch to make a decision that changed the course of his life, here on earth, and in eternity. In this chapter I'm going to be your Phillip.

This eunuch was reading what he knew to be the book of the prophet Isaiah, but he didn't understand what he was reading. The word of God is our spiritual food, and understanding it helps us to grow, change, and get closer to God. Carbohydrates, protein, fats, fiber, and water are part of the physical food we eat, and understanding them will help your body be closer to the level of health and fitness you desire.

Understanding Carbohydrates

Carbohydrates are the type of foods that provide the main source of energy for all bodily functions. Everyday activities and muscular exertion (from exercise) cause a rapid depletion of carbohydrates. As depletion occurs, the body sends us signals in the form of cravings so that the energy source can be replaced; thus our craving to consume carbohydrates such as bread, rice, pasta, and sweets is normal and is a natural response to the body's need for energy. Where we go wrong is that we overeat and eat too much of the wrong type of carbohydrates.

Another important function of carbohydrates is that they help regulate the digestion and utilization of protein and fat. When carbohydrates are consumed, the body breaks them down to sugar glucose, which is absorbed by the body and used for energy. If the body produces too much glucose, the glucose will be stored in the form of glycogen (discussed in Chapter 5) in the liver and muscles and fat cells.

There are two types of carbohydrates: simple and complex.

Simple carbohydrates, also called simple sugars, are found in foods such as fruits and are often found in processed foods and anything with refined sugar, and are most easily digested by the body. Fruits are excellent as a quick pick-me-up, but they usually are not good enough to keep most people satisfied for long periods of time. I usually have fruit before or during a workout or in the middle of the day when I feel tired, because it digests fast and gives me an instant source of energy.

This simple sugar has a positive impact on the body and can help you manage your weight.

On the other hand, the refined sugar and starches found in processed carbohydrates, candies, and other sweets have a negative impact on your ability to lose and maintain your weight. They create a rapid spike in blood sugar levels (as discussed in Chapter 5), which causes the body to produce a high level of insulin, which rapidly moves the sugar out of the blood and into the cells. This causes the blood sugar level to decrease rapidly, producing a carbohydrate craving to replace that which was depleted. Consumption of processed foods as a main source of carbohydrates stimulates within the body a constant craving for sugary foods,[46] causing many people to overeat in an effort to satisfy the craving.

Complex carbohydrates are found in almost all plant-based foods and usually take longer for the body to digest. They are most commonly found in bread, rice, and pasta, and in vegetables. These types of carbohydrate, specifically if they are whole grain products, keep us satisfied longer, and do not cause the rapid rise in blood sugar levels that causes a spike in insulin production. When consumed in the appropriate amounts, complex carbs can help you maintain and lose weight by keeping you energized and providing the body with the nutrients it needs. You don't need to avoid carbohydrates; you need to eat the right types in the right amounts.

Because the consumption of carbohydrates is an important part of making energy to the body available, no-carb and low-carb diets can be very dangerous and have an adverse effect on your ability to lose weight and maintain weight. Not eating enough carbohydrates is just as bad as eating too many. Most people will experience weight loss on no-carb or low-carb diets, but the results are usually temporary, and can have damaging effects on your body and your mind as you try to maintain this type of lifestyle. Absence of an adequate amount of carbohydrates in the body causes loss of energy (making it hard to work out) and a breakdown of lean muscle tissue, which as explained earlier, slows down the metabolism, causes uncontrollable cravings, and causes weight regain

---

[46] Cynthia Conde: Bridal boot camp- Look Fabulous on your big day pg 24 (Running Press Book Publishing, Philadelphia, PA 2004)

after a return to normal eating. It's simply not worth it; you're in this to reach and maintain your fitness goals for life.

Some of you are probably wondering, "But isn't this what body builders and fitness competitors do?" The answer is yes, but understand that they deplete themselves of carbs only in the few weeks or days leading right up to the competition. The majority of fitness competitors and body builders have a more balanced way of eating during the rest of the year, and go through dieting on and off seasons. You really can't compare the diet of a professional body builder or fitness competitor to that of the average person.

So What Are the Best Types of Carbs to Eat?

Whether they are complex or simple carbohydrates, not all carbohydrates are created equal; there are some that are better for us than others. The *glycemic index,* or GI,[47] is the method most commonly used to determine which carbohydrates are best. The glycemic index ranks carbohydrates on a scale of 0 to 100, based on the extent they raise blood sugar and insulin levels. Blood sugar levels, also called blood glucose, refer to how much sugar is in the blood. As discussed earlier, high spikes in blood sugar cause insulin levels to increase, this rapidly ushers the sugar out of the blood causing hunger. The glycemic index measures how much your blood glucose increases after eating foods containing carbohydrates.

High-GI foods, 70 and higher, make blood sugar and insulin level rise fast. These foods "fill you quickly and give you a fast burst of energy,[48]" but they leave you feeling hungry and tired shortly thereafter. White bread and certain forms of rice and pasta and other processed foods are common examples, and are what many nutritionists consider "bad carbs."

Foods between 55 and 70 are considered medium-GI foods. Low-GI foods (less than 55) produce a small rise in blood sugar and insulin levels.

---

[47] "What Is the Glycemic Index?" www.wisegeek.com.
[48] Ibid

These foods fill you up without causing a rapid rise in blood sugar. Blood sugar rises "slowly and steadily," causing you to feel fuller for a longer period of time, while also supplying the body with "continuous energy." These are considered the "good carbs" and are found in whole grain foods, fruits, and vegetables.

High glycemic carbs are usually good for those who need quick energy: athletes are a good example. But for most people, especially those trying to lose weight, choosing low glycemic foods are the way to go because they make you feel fuller longer, making it less likely that you will overeat. But remember, choosing low glycemic carbs is not a license to eat as much as you want. Paying attention to what you eat is as important as paying attention to how much you eat.

For myself, I find that although fruits are low-GI foods, because some of them like apples or oranges are simple carbohydrates and digest faster, they give me a burst of energy. If it's lunchtime and I'm hungry, instead of starving myself through my workout, I'll have a fruit and then eat my lunch afterward. That way I get the energy I need without feeling a little sluggish because I just ate a normal meal. Not placing something in the body before a workout is like expecting your car to drive 10 miles without gas; the car won't get far and neither will your body exercising on an empty stomach.

A list of foods and their glycemic index level contains the most common foods that most people eat. A list can be fo*und on the web by typing the words "glycemic Index" into your search browser.*

Understanding Protein

Protein is necessary for growth and development of body tissue, and the formation of hormones that control many bodily functions such as growth and metabolic rate. Each gram of protein, as you learned earlier, contains about 4 calories. Under normal circumstances where there is enough carbohydrate and fat in one's diet, the body does not use protein as a source of energy, but when people carb deplete (as suggested in many popular no-carb diets), the body will use protein as a source of energy, leaving less available for the development of body tissues and other functions. This essentially causes the breakdown of muscle tissue in the body. And since muscle tissue burns more energy than fat tissue, there will be an eventual slow down in the metabolic rate.

There are two types of proteins: complete and incomplete. Foods are considered *complete proteins* when they contain all essential amino acids. Amino acids are the "building blocks" of the body. They build cells, repair tissue, and form antibodies that help fight off bacteria and viruses.[49] Meat, milk, and eggs are considered complete proteins. *Incomplete proteins* are found in grains, legumes, seeds, nuts, and vegetables; these foods lack one or more essential amino acids needed to provide a complete source of protein. The daily recommended amount of protein intake is 20–25 percent of your total calorie intake. If you're a meat eater, you probably have enough protein in your diet. Although lean proteins are good for us, it is possible to over consume. Over consumption of protein especially in the form of meat can have a stool hardening effect, making excretion more difficult, and could even cause the colon to be blocked. I would say that in general women should eat about 3 to 4 ounces of meat, and men from 4 to 6. Dietary intake of protein or any other nutrient for that matter should always relate back to the health and fitness goals of the individual. For vegetarians, meals containing complete proteins can be made by combining foods from the grain category with foods from the legumes or seed and nut category[50]:

Grains: brown rice, wheat pasta, buckwheat, breads, barley
Legumes: beans, lentils, peas, peanuts, soy products
Vegetable: broccoli, cabbage, asparagus, Brussels sprout, collard greens
Nuts: walnuts, cashews, sunflower seeds

It is recommended that sedentary adults consume about 0.8 gm/kg/day of protein. Physically active adults need about 1.2 grams of protein per pound of lean muscle tissue per day. This is calculated by:

---

[49] Reference Guide For Amino Acids
   www.realtime.net/anr/aminoacd.html
[50] Hinger, Jolynn eds; Apex FintenssManuel pg16. (published by The Apex Group, Camarilla CA 2001)

Weight (in pounds) divided by 2.2 = ___ kg
Weight in kg x 1.2gm protein= _____gm

I want to stress to you once again that diets low in carbohydrates and high in protein can be very dangerous. Consuming very little carbohydrates and very high amounts of protein over a long period of time, causes protein to be used for energy rather than for maintaining and building muscle.

Now some of you may know or have read that body builders and fitness competitors believe in high-protein diets. Yes this true, but most only increase their protein intake in the final weeks before a competition because they are trying to reach a very low body-fat level. The majority of body builders and fitness competitors follow a more balanced diet during their off season.

When the famous Atkins Diet first came out, I, like many others, was pulled into the low-carb crave, even though I was already thin and in good shape. But I was so obsessed. I had that little lower stomach area that didn't seem to want to go away, no matter what I did. So I thought that the Atkins Diet was the answer. So I threw away all I had learned about balance and moderation that had made me successful, and just went on an extreme diet. Well, I did for nine weeks. All the while I was still running and weight training. Then one day while in my room, my body started to shake. I realized that I was involved in all these activities that required energy, and I was giving my body nothing but protein and fat. I also noticed that I had more muscle soreness than usual, all a result, I'm sure, of the breakdown occurring in my muscles. Without the right type of carbohydrates I was breaking my body down. There are many who swear by a no-carb diet, my advice is that the best path to lifetime success in the nutritional area of your life is balance and moderation.

Understanding Fat

Fats are the most concentrated form of food energy; each gram of fat contains 9 calories. Fat provides the body with more calories per gram than protein or carbohydrates, which only have 4 calories per gram. Fat is a necessary nutrient for cell membrane and hormone development. The fat cells surrounding the body organs are what help insulate us. It is the fat in food that makes us feel satisfied, so it is important to eat the right type of fat in the appropriate amounts. In general, dietary fat intake can be between 15 to 20 percent of total calorie intake. Good fats are found in lean cuts of meat and mono- and polyunsaturated fat foods such as avocados, nuts, oil (olive, canola, peanut, sesame), and the omega oils found in flaxseed oil and fish and shell fish. Bad fats include saturated and trans fats. Saturated and trans fats are found in cooking oils such as butter and shortening and are used in fried foods, processed foods like cookies, crackers, cakes, chips, store-bought bread, and many soups. And let's not forget fast foods; not to worry, though, in a later chapter I will show you how to fit fast food into a healthy lifestyle. Trans fats are also found in stick margarine and nondairy creamers.

Trans Fats: The New Bad Fat

Trans fats are our new worst enemy in the battle to stave off excess weight. Trans fat are found mainly in processed foods and are listed not in the fat content of food labels but within the ingredients. A trans fat is a mixture of fats and oils that are hydrogenated (combined) as a way to extend the shelf life of food. Trans fats are more dangerous than saturated fats because they raise cholesterol levels significantly higher than saturated fats and can contribute to higher levels of weight gain, making it hard to lose or maintain weight.

Previously, the FDA had not required food companies to list trans fat content on their nutritional labels, but beginning in January 2006, the FDA approved a measure that would require all food companies to list trans fat content in their products. Manufactures have used trans fat in their products because it extends the shelf life of products. Many companies have begun to stop using trans fats to make their products, as consumers are becoming more aware of how dangerous they are. But you must sill beware, because although many food labels list zero trans fats on the nutritional label, looking at the ingredients tells another story. Products with trans fats in them contain "shortening" and/or a "partially hydrogenated" type oil. So despite what the labels says, what's listed in the ingredients portion of the food label tells the whole story.

The amount of trans fats in a product generally increase the fat content by 3 grams or more. As a result, many products marketed as fat-free or low-fat may in fact contain high levels of fat that their makers are not required to report to us. So—buyer beware!

It is important to understand that a diet with very little to no saturated or trans fats is one of the keys to losing and maintaining weight loss. But don't avoid fats altogether. Use mono- and polyunsaturated which are better for the body.

A major reason why poly- and monounsaturated fats are considered good fats and better for the body is that these fats melt at a lower temperature than saturated and trans fats. With regards to losing and maintaining weight, this means that we don't have to produce as much energy (elevation in body temperature due to exercise and other activities) in order to burn the calories(convert the fat into readily usable energy) that come from these types of fats. Saturated and trans fats melt at significantly higher room temperatures, which means that it takes a lot more work (energy expenditure on our parts) in order to burn off the calories from these fats.

Understanding Fiber

Foods rich in fiber provide bulk, which makes you feel full. Fiber can be found in many fruits, vegetables, and whole grains. The other benefit of fiber is that it prevents constipation and helps establish regular bowel movements, lowers the risk of colon cancer, and reduces heart artery disease. Twenty-five grams per day is the recommended daily allowance of fiber.

Understanding Water

Adequate water consumption is essential for converting fat to energy. The recommended daily intake is 8 glasses or 64ounces a day, but 96 ounces or three quarts of water per day is a better goal to strive for. If your goal is fat loss and you are participating in a fat loss program, it is recommended that you drink an additional 8 ounces of water for every

25 pounds over your ideal weight.[51] I drink about a gallon of water of day. Drinking the adequate amount of water benefits your body in a number of ways.[52] It helps to improve liver function, which increases the amount of fat used for energy, can help suppress the appetite, increases the metabolism, and alleviates water retention (loss of water weight). Water is also important for maintaining normal bowel movements, which should be about two to three times per day, and flushes toxins out of the body.

Water and Your Workout

During your workout, it is important to stay hydrated. This can be done by drinking at least six ounces of water every ten to fifteen minutes. If your workout exceeds ninety minutes, use a sports drink that contains less than 7 percent carbohydrates (check the percentage of carbohydrates on the nutritional label). Also hydration keeps the body energized. As we work out the blood (the body's transport system), has to work much faster to deliver oxygen to working muscles. If the body is not hydrated enough the blood is more placid or sticky, and move slower through the body, causing the premature unset a fatigue. But if the body is properly hydrated the blood has a higher level of liquidity, and can therefore move faster through the vessel to deliver much needed oxygen to working muscles.

Understanding Sodium

For those whose goal is to lose weight, it is very important to watch sodium intake. Besides causing the risk of developing high blood pressure, too much sodium in your diet can also cause you to retain a lot of water (be bloated). Too much salt retains water, and water retains fat. Chips, frozen entrees (even healthy ones), salad dressings, tomato and pasta sauces, gravys and canned foods such as soups usually contain high amounts of sodium. Pre-marinated and deli meats also have high sodium contents. One slice of deli meat can contain as much as 1000 milligrams of salt. I know that in the real world we may not be able to

---

[51] Ibid pg23

[52] Ibid pg 24

always avoid high sodium products. The best defense against salt induced water retention, believe it of not is to drink more water. Water will help you body to flush out excess sodium, and help you maintain a healthy sodium balance.

Tips for Reducing Sodium Intake

If you are really truly interested in having some solid guidelines about sodium intake, provided here are some of the rules I thumb that I use when I food shop. When selecting canned foods, I reach for products with 300 grams of sodium or less per serving. For soups, I either choose the low-sodium brand or buy the ones with 500 or less per serving.

Before eating deli meats, boil them for two to three minutes whenever possible. This will remove some of the salt. Replace the taste with low-cal mayo, mustard, or low-fat cheese. All have salt in them but not as much.

Put canned beans and veggies in a strainer and rinse them for two minutes or so. Remember to drink your water. This will flush excess sodium out of your body.

Be aware that when ordering out, most of the food will be high in sodium, so make sure to drink some water with your meal.

Now that you have a better understanding of what is going into your body, you have been equipped to take control of your situation. In the same way that God has prepared you to function in other areas in your life, he is now preparing you to change unhealthy eating habits. Your negative relationship with food, whether you eat too much or too little, has now therefore been destroyed. God gives us knowledge, and with knowledge comes wisdom. You can now make wise decisions about what goes into your body. After Phillip explained to the eunuch what he was reading, he understood, and when he understood, he got baptized (he changed). The wisdom that he received from understanding the knowledge he was reading caused him to accept Jesus as his personal Lord and savior. And praise God, because he has granted this to you as an expression of his love and his desire for you to have as complete an understanding of the foods you eat, as possible.

Chapter 9

Eat More, Weigh Less

"….let God transforms you into a new
person by changing the way you think. Then
you will know God's will for you, which
is good, and pleasing, and perfect"
(Romans 12:2)

It may be hard to believe that you can eat more and weigh less, but it's very possible. When I think about this concept, what comes to mind is how reading God's word (the food that feeds the spirit), has allowed me to get rid of and be delivered from a lot of emotional baggage. When I study the word of God on my own, I don't always read the whole chapter at the same time. I read a set of verses at a time, and then I write in my Bible study journal the lesson being taught and my thoughts. The writing part helps me to digest what I just read and to process it. Then a little while later, I read on and do the same thing again. I have found that reading the word very often but in small doses over the day makes it easier for me to understand what the Lord wants me to see, and I don't become overwhelmed by trying to get it all at once. Recording what I read, my thoughts, and any insight the Holy Spirit may have given me allows me to also review what I learned from time to time so that it stays fresh in my mind. This has allowed me to become less and less spiritually weighed down. I eat more to weigh less because, it easier for me to digest and process God's word, enabling me to understand enough to apply the word to every area of my life.

It is in this same way that I have found that by eating several small meals throughout the day, I was able to lose a lot of weight. The concept behind eating five to six small meals a day as opposed to eating three big meals a day is that eating often (and making the right food choices) keeps the blood sugar level more stable. As we discussed before, dips in blood sugar levels cause cravings for sugary, fatty foods and white starches (the result of carbohydrate depletion). The foods we crave during these energy dips are also the result of our upbringing and our emotional connection to food.

I can show you how to counteract the biological aspect by showing how to form the habit of eating smaller meals more often. But you have to make a commitment between God and you to deal with your emotional connection to food. In prayer, ask the Lord to show you your habits, and ask him to show you why you have them (where did they all begin, and what's going on underneath it all), and then tell him you want to be delivered from any unhealthy emotional connections you have with food. Ask God where you can go to be delivered, and while you wait, you yourself bind up that emotional connection in the name of Jesus (Matt. 18:18). Ask him to give you a support network of fellow Christians you can pray with. Believe me, there are evil spiritual forces behind your unhealthy eating habits. But as the word says, we don't fight against the flesh but against wicked spirits (Ephesians 6:12). Behind that unhealthy emotional connection is an evil spirit manipulating you, feeding into it, and influencing situations and circumstances that cause you to give in.

But maybe you feel that this is not true for you. Maybe not, but ask God anyway if you do have any unhealthy emotional connections to food. It won't hurt just to ask.

Biologically speaking, smaller meals make it easier for the body to break down and digest food. The key is to eat every three hours. Eating every three hours also helps to stabilize your blood sugar level. So not only are you eating smaller meals, but you are eating them closer together. I don't know about you, but as a person who loves to eat, I was more than happy that I could eat every three hours.

I found that with myself and my clients, eating this way curbs the tendencies to overeat during the day by building snacks into the day. Yes, you can have your cake and eat it, too. The best way to get started is to sit down and write down an approximate schedule of when you will eat. Now you might not be able to eat at that time exactly every day, but it provides you with a plan of action.

For example, here is a sample of my schedule:

My day starts at 4:15 each day. I spend the first thirty minutes in prayer.

Meal #1: 4:45 AM; for me a morning snack, usually 8 ounces of fat-free milk mixed with a scoop of chocolate-flavored powder protein and a teaspoon of flaxseed oil.
Meal#2: 8:00 AM (Breakfast)
Meal#3: 11:00 AM or 12:00 PM (Lunch)
Meal#4: 3:00 PM (Snack)
Meal#5: 6:00 PM (Dinner)
Meal#6: 9:00 PM(Snack); because I usually like to eat something sweet after dinner, it might be a fruit or a yogurt or 8-ounces of cereal ½ cup of fat-free milk, almond, or hazelnut milk (4 oz.), or ½ cup of frozen yogurt with some berries. I might even have a decaf skim milk latte.

You can choose to have five actual meals, if you want, like a small sandwich instead of a snack.

The Benefits

Eating smaller meals every three hours helps the body to digest food more efficiently, allows calories to be burned more quickly, and causes less of what we eat to be stored as fat. The fewer calories we store as fat, the less we look fat. Also, eating this way will complement the commitment you have already made to become physically active and make better food choices, helping you to reach your goals faster. The greatest benefit is you get to eat more often and still lose weight.

Now if your problem is not to lose weight, but to gain weight, eating this way will force you to eat more. This will also help once a day/twice a day big-meal eaters to began to break down some of the stored fat within the body. Once you are giving your body energy (food) in smaller doses more often, it will be biologically less necessary for the body to overstore calories. The regularity of your eating will send the body the signal that it will be constantly reenergized, giving the body the green light to empty out fat stores. Irregular and erratic eating habits make the body less willing to release its fat stores.

Common Issues

I Don't Have Time to Eat Every Three Hours

Sure you do, it depends on what you're eating. Most of us have a time we eat breakfast, lunch, and dinner each day, so just add easy snacks, like a fruit, a yogurt, an energy or protein bar (energy bars are usually good before a workout, or in the afternoon when you feel a little tired). All it takes is a five-minute break. I always carry something in my purse just in case.

I Feel Like I'm Eating Too Much

If you calculate what you eat just once or twice a day, you'll find that you may already be eating more than you should. Now you're going to start eating smarter by taking those same calories or less and just spreading them out more evenly throughout the day.

Things to Consider

- Watch your portions.

- Based on your schedule, most people find it better to make lunch the biggest of the meals.

- Veggies should be a part of lunch and dinner (remember that corn, carrots, and sweet peas are starches).

- Choose steamed over fried.

- Eat one serving of a complex carb that has a low to medium glycemic index with at least two of your meals. I do this for the three main meals. Remember, low glycemic carbs help stabilize your blood sugar level.

- Remember to watch out for those liquid calories in juices and sodas.

- Choose water, and low- to no-calories drinks like diet soda and diet juice drinks.

- Choose healthy mono- and polyunsaturated fats and/or use only the serving size of the oil or dressing (such as mayo), nuts, or cheese you use. And choose to have one or the other and not both.

- Don't skip meals and then try to make up for it later!

- Overloading on calories will only cause the body to store more fat. Not eating enough will keep your metabolic rate low.

OK. When will you eat tomorrow, and what will you eat based on what you know so far? Write it down in a little notebook

You can plan your meals in advance in the same way you plan your daily schedule—in fact do it at the same time. I found it helpful to keep a food journal. Not only did it show my bad habits, it made me more aware of what I was putting into my body, and gave me something to look back on. Much the same way, writing down what I study from the word and my thoughts makes me more aware of what God is saying to me and gives me something to look back on when I need to refresh my memory.

Prayer:

Dear heavenly Father you are a ever-present help in a time of need.
I ask your dear Lord to help me be committed to tracking what
I eat each day. I may have tried and failed to do this in the past, but
Now Lord, I'm asking you to transform my mind and the way I think
about food. Thank you Lord, I am ever grateful to you for your love and
support. In Jesus name Amen.

Chapter 10

Vitamins, Minerals, and Supplements

"I baptize with water, those who repent of their
sins and return to God, but someone coming
soon greater that I- am…. He will baptize you
with the Holy Spirit and fire"- John the Baptist
(Matthew 3:11)

In the world of Christianity there are thousands of books that cover a wide variety of subjects. These books operate as tools that teach us how to apply God's word in different areas of our lives or just give us a better understanding of the book itself. I have read a lot myself, and there is nothing that I have read that has not given me a deeper understanding of God's will, purpose, and plan for my life. But as intriguing as these books are, they could never replace or act as a substitute for reading and studying the Bible itself. These books are only a supplement to the word of God in helping me to reach my goal of developing a closer fellowship with him. John the Baptist baptized people but he made it very clear, that he was just a substitute, a stand- in to prepare people for the coming of the messiah. The Baptism that John the Baptist performed was in no way, shape, or form meant to take the place of the greater one to be given to us by the Messiah himself. It is in this same manner that multivitamins and mineral supplements are not a replacements for food but are "designed to complement your best diet efforts"[53] to achieve the level of optimal nutrition that corresponds with your fitness goal. In other words, vitamins and minerals are like your sidekick.

Multivitamin and mineral supplements are beneficial because they help to support and maintain cellular functions on different levels, including helping the body to shed excess fat, and prompting repair and recovery. Exercise and the resulting physical adaptations such as gaining lean muscle increase the usage of nutrients by the body, and

---

[53] Ibid pg 33

multivitamins and mineral supplements replace these nutrients without adding calories, picking up where food leaves off.

Realistically, one would have to consume large quantities of food to meet the minimum standards of nutritional adequacy. This is counterproductive, particularly for reducing body fat. Reducing body fat requires maintaining your intake so that you are always burning more than what you are taking in. At the same time, increases in physical activity levels create the need for more nutrients. Multivitamin and mineral supplements are the best way to provide nutrients to the body and maintain your goal of a specific level of food intake.

Nutrient Delivery

How well a multivitamin works in providing your body the nutrients it needs depends on how the nutrient, once in the body, is delivered to the cells.[54] Most formulas are digested so quickly by the body that they throw all the nutrients at the cell at once. Naturally, the cells can't take them in all at once, which usually results in a large part of the nutrients never being absorbed and used. They simply pass through the system and come out in your urine. Timed-released formulas are better because nutrients are designed to be delivered to the cells over a period of eight to twelve hours, allowing the body to get the full benefit of the nutrient.

It is also important to pay attention to the dosage recommendation and in some cases, start off with half that for the first few days to get the body use to taking it. Not following labeling directions and/or not starting off slow could reduce the overall effectiveness of the nutrient for achieving optimal nutrition.

Generally Recommended Supplements

A multivitamin, calcium (especially for women), and an antioxidant are recommended across the board for all fitness goals and levels. There are more sports and weight-training-specific supplements that are

---

[54] Ibid pg 34-36

commonly used such as creatine, glutamine, and branch chain amino acids.

A multivitamin is useful for supplying the body with vitamins and minerals that are being obtained directly from food. The brand or type of multivitamin one uses really depends on individual need. An athletic person, the heavy weight trainer, and a person into just general fitness, all have different needs based on level of activity, age, and gender. When if comes to multivitamin formulas I do believe that liquid is better than pill form, because is more readily digestible. Calcium helps to build strong bones and helps muscle function. Antioxidants "are vitamins, minerals, and other nutrients that protect and repair cells from damage caused by free radicals."[55] Free radicals are by-products of normal processes that take place in your body (such as the burning of sugars for energy and the release of digestive enzymes to break down food), and when the body breaks down certain medicines through pollutants.[56] So we are always exposed to them.

Creatine supplements help to increase "high intensity athletic performance"[57] Glutamine is a supplement that aid in muscle recovery and can be taken before or after heavy training. Glutamine can help to reduce muscle soreness. Branch- chain amino supplements acids are a group of amino acid that are taken to help maintain muscle tissue that is subjected to intense exercise. A diet that contains animal protein usually provides the necessary amount of BCAA's for most people. For those who work out intensely, BCAA's can help prevent muscle loss, and spur muscle gain.

Meal-Replacement and Snack Supplements

Other types of supplements include meal-replacement protein powders, shakes, bars, and healthy energy and snack bars. These are the types of supplements that can be incorporated into a five to six day meal plan. They are a great because they make it easier to have a meal without having to cook, and they are available almost everywhere you go. You

---

[55] http://www.webmd.com
[56] Ibid
[57] Http://www.wikipedia.com

can have three actual food meals and then add two to three shakes or bars in between. But also always remember to pay attention to calorie, fat, sugar content, and protein content (10 to 20 grams of protein in a shake or bar is generally good).

Energy bars tend to have high amounts of sugar, so these are best consumed before a workout or as an afternoon pick-me-up. Generally, 10 to 15 grams of sugar is OK, if you are not consuming high amounts of sugar elsewhere in your diet. Protein bars are good to consume after weight training. Generally, the bar you choose should contain carbohydrates (on average 25 to 30 grams) so that the protein will be used for muscle building and not for energy (as discussed in Chapter 8). But they can also be consumed before a workout to supply the body with pre-workout nutrients. My first meal of the day is a protein shake(a mixture of a chocolate protein powder, 1 cup of almond milk, and 1teaspoon of flaxseed oil) right before I go to the gym. Some protein powders can have a bloating effect- Especially for women. I suggest trying a protein powder formulated specifically for your needs. Not all powders are created equal. There are protein supplements just for women and men, for general health, and for athletes and body builders. This is a time to really asses what it is you are trying to achieve and set out to understand what supplements are best for you. I personally found that whey protein products while they gave me great results, always made me feel bloated. After months of experimenting I found a protein that was lactose free, and not made of whey protein.

Chapter 11

Fitting Fast Food into a Healthy Lifestyle

"Everything is permissible for me—but not
everything is beneficial. Everything is permissible
for me—but I will not be mastered by anything."
(1 Corinthians 6:12)

It is permissible to eat any kind of food you like, but not everything you eat is beneficial for your body. Fast foods are, for the most part, very unhealthy. The high sodium and fat contents possess very little benefit in terms of what is considered good nutrition. If fast food is too much of a significant part of what is being consumed each day, it becomes a barrier that prevents us from experiencing the fullness of health that God wants for us. Eating fast food has so many negative impacts on overall health that it can come to master how the body looks and feels. God says to you today as the Apostle Paul said; do not be mastered by anything. Eating fast food in moderation and learning how to make the right choice will release you from being a slave of poor health. And remember thinness does not equate to healthiness, so no matter what you weigh, over consuming fast food can be dangerous to your health.

Learning how to fit fast food into a healthy lifestyle can help you to attain and maintain your desired level of fitness. I agree with most people in the world of nutrition and fitness that the consumption of fast food has become a dangerous epidemic in American society and is a leading cause for obesity among both children and adults. As an experienced nutritional adviser, I believe that it is always best, whenever possible, to prepare and carry your own meals, but I also understand that this is not always possible. It is therefore better to learn how to consume fast food, and how to dine out in moderation as opposed to attempting to cut out these foods completely. If you apply these concepts no matter where you eat, you will always be in control, which will help keep you on track. I know it's possible, because I do it myself. The bottom line is portion control. Here are some general suggestions about how to make the best food choices in different types of restaurants and fast-food places.

First, there are several things that you should be aware of in fast-food restaurants.

Frying can triple the fat content. Whenever possible, choose baked, broiled, and grilled menu items. Mayonnaise and salad dressing add major calories. Always ask for low-fat/fat-free alternatives. If there are none, ask for dressing on the side and use sparingly or ask for olive oil (a healthy fat. But remember even if you chose a healthy fat don't overdo it; pour the oil into your spoon and then pour it into your salad. Also choose condiments like mustard, ketchup, and salsa. Especially if your meal has more than one source of fat, be careful with cheese. It is common for salads to contain cheese, bacon, nuts, and oil/dressing. Make a choice which one you want the most. Croutons are a deep-fried caloric wasteland that can be lethal to your waistline. Be careful about liquid wasted calories. Juice and regular soda don't fill you up; in fact, they can make you eat more. Drink water or diet beverages instead. Watch out for portion distortion. Don't be the victim of the supersize, which can add 500–2000 calories to your meal. In fact, I would urge you to get the child-size meal and have a side salad and some fruit as a dessert. If you have not waited until you are extremely hungry to eat, a child-size meal and some fruit can satisfy you. Many burger chains now have dollar menus that offer smaller versions of their main menu options. A dollar menu chicken sandwich is much smaller then a regular-sized one, making it the better option. Portion distortion is most rampant in diners and restaurants, so when eating in these places, ask the server to bring you a take-out container with your order. Put half the food in the container and place it off to the side to take home, and eat what's left on your plate. Nine times out of ten most people end up throwing the food away after they refrigerate it. Congratulations, you just saved yourself 500 calories or more. Also watch out for too many starches. On regular-sized meals, having the burger and fries (having bread and potatoes in the same meal), is a lot of calories to consume. As discussed earlier, starches, which are carbohydrates, are the body's chief source of energy. Any leftover that the body does not need is converted into fat—which most of us wish to avoid. So choose the bread or the rice, or the potato, and so on.

Pandora N. Kinard

Some Other Things You Can Do

Going Light to Make Your Latte or Coffee Right

Enjoy your favorite latte or coffee with skim milk and/or fat-free half and half. Also choose sugar-free syrup to flavor your coffee. But if you must have it your way, choose the small. You will be surprised to find that you don't need to have as much as you thought to satisfy your craving. You walk away getting what you want, absent of the guilt. You get to have your cake and eat it, too.

Make It Special

Make eating fast food, whenever possible, a once a week or special occasion event; that way you will learn to appreciate it more. If you have been good all week (and don't lie to yourself, because it only hurts you, remember you made your commitment to be healthy with yourself and God), then go ahead and dig in on a Saturday or Sunday for one meal only; whether it be breakfast, lunch, or dinner. I have one cheat meal a week on Saturdays. And I never feel bad about it, especially if I know that I made all of the right choices all week long, out of what was available to me.

Here are some moderate-calorie food choices from the most common fast-food places. Please keep in mind that almost all fast foods are high in fat and sodium. The key again is to enjoy them in moderation.

McDonald's:

Breakfast
Plain English muffin (150)
Egg McMuffin (300 Calories)
Sausage Breakfast Burrito (290)
Hot Cakes without syrup or butter; one order (280)

Burgers
Plain hamburger (280)
Plain McGrilled Classic Chicken (250)
McLean Deluxe (340)
Wraps: Grilled Chicken snack wrap (260)

Dessert
Hot caramel low-fat sundae (310)
Strawberry low-fat frozen yogurt (240)
Vanilla low-fat frozen yogurt (120)
Apple bran muffin (180)
Low Fat Yogurt Parfait (160)

Burger King:

Breakfast
Croissan'wich with egg and cheese (350). Be mindful that this item has 24 grams of fat. And skip the sausage option on this one. The meat adds another 260 calories.
Hash brown; one (220)

Burgers
Plain hamburger (330)

Arby's:

Breakfast
Blueberry muffin
Hot chocolate, small (110)

Sandwiches
Light roast beef deluxe (296)
Junior roast beef (324)
Light roast chicken deluxe (267)
Light roast turkey deluxe (260)
ham and cheese (359)

Potato, plain (355)

Soups
Lumberjack mixed vegetable (90)
Old-fashioned chicken noodle (80)

Subway Sandwich and Subs:

Breakfast
Western Egg Breakfast Sandwich (300)

Subs
4-inch round

Ham (209)
Roast beef (233)
Seafood and crab with light mayo (232)

6-inch subs under 6grams of fat. (300–450). On wheat, without cheese or mayo. Cheese and mayonnaise add 200–400 more calories.

Taco Bell: (these choices have 10grams of fat or less)

Light bean burrito (330)
Light Burrito Supreme (350)
Light Chicken Burrito (290)
Light Chicken Burrito Supreme (410)
Light Chicken Soft Taco (180)
Light Seven Layer Burrito (440)
Light Soft Taco (180)
Light Soft Taco Supreme (200)
Light Taco Salad without chips (330)

Light Taco Supreme (160)

Side orders
Seasoned rice (110)

KFC:
Original Recipe Chicken Breast and small mashed potatoes (500)
Small barbecue baked beans (132)
Garden rice (75)
Green beans (36)
Red beans and rice (114)

Pizza Hut:
Two slices of thin crust:
With reduced fat cheese (410)
Veggie Lovers (372)

Hand tossed pizza:
Ham, two slices (426)
Veggie Lovers (432)

Wendy's:
Plain potato (310)
Small chili (190)
Large chili (290)
Saltine crackers (25)

Boston Market:
Meatloaf (310) with potato salad (add another 200)
Marinated Grilled Chicken Sandwich (470 without cheese or mayo)

Denny's:

Breakfast
Bagel, plain (230)
English muffin, Plain (150)
Hash browns (164)
Oatmeal (70)
Buttermilk pancakes, plain (410)

Pandora N. Kinard

Soup
Chicken noodle soup (45)
Split pea soup (231)
Veggie beef soup (60)

Grilled chicken sandwich (439)
Small mashed potatoes (60)
Small baked potato (115)
Spaghetti w/tomato sauce (600)
Top sirloin steak (entree only; 223)
Turkey entrée, no gravy (505)

Dunkin' Donuts:
Bagels
Plain (230)
Cinnamon and raisin (230)
Onion (210)
Egg White flatbread sandwich (300)
Multigrain bagel (360)
Drinks
Skim milk latte, medium (120)

Muffins
Low-fat apple spice (220)
Low-fat banana (240)
Low-fat cranberry orange (230)

Baskin-Robbins:
Mocha cappuccino blast bar (120)

Cones
Sugar (60)
Waffle (146)

Fat-free dairy desserts, ½ cup
Chocolate vanilla twist (100)
Jamoca Swirl (110)
Just Peachy (100)

Frozen yogurt, ½ cup
Low-fat chocolate and vanilla (120)
Nonfat Dutch and strawberry (100)
Nonfat vanilla (110)

Light dairy desserts, ½ cup
Espresso and cream (110)
Praline (120)

No sugar added, ½ cup
Jamoca Swiss almond (100)
Red raspberry sorbet

Toppings
Butterscotch (100)
Strawberry (60)

TCBY, ½ cup:
Nonfat frozen yogurt, flavors (110)
No sugar added/nonfat frozen flavors (80)
Regular frozen yogurt, flavors (130)
Sorbet (100)

The Cheat Day

Having one cheat meal per week is an important component of reaching and maintaining you fitness goal. By having one cheat meal a week, you have something to motivate you to eat healthy. Your cheat meal can be any day of the week and can be planned around any special events. I usually have mine on Saturday or Sunday. I think Sunday is better because then I just start a new week on Monday. Saturday night cheat meals can sometimes spill into Sunday if you're not careful.

Your cheat meal can be whatever you want to eat, as long as you have been good the whole week. Make sure you are being honest with yourself about this; don't forget—God is watching also.

Chapter 12

Putting It All Together

The key to your success in this area of your life is allowing the word of God to reach down into your spirit so that it may govern and help you apply all the principles and concepts that you have learned. Absent of the word of God, the soul (thoughts and emotions) will rule in this area. It is what's in your sprits that will break the strongholds of the devil in this area of you life, allowing you to regain control over your health. Taking hold of the spiritual aspect causes a better understanding of what is going on in the soul (how and why you relate to food the way you do and why you don't exercise). The transformation of the soul by way of the spirit (which holds the word), will release you to receive and apply the concepts expressed because it changes the way you think.

As expressed in the beginning of this book, being healthy provides a strong physical vessel for the Lord's use. So if you can't find any other reason to start eating right and exercising, think about it along these lines. Know that God cares about your body because it is a living sacrifice, and it matters how the sacrifice is presented and the condition it's in. The greatest thing we can do is give the Lord our best; he is worthy of it.

Proper nutrition, cardiovascular training, weight training, dietary support (supplements), undergirded by the word of God, will propel you toward the right level of health, because it moves beyond the vanity of it. If vanity was enough to motivate us, everyone would be eating right and exercising.

To Sum It All Up

Above all else, pray and praise and worship: I don't care how much you have learned, it is this that will allow to you to cross the abyss into a healthier lifestyle and achieve your fitness goals. Because believe me when I tell you, any time a child of God tries to do something positive, the devil is plotting and scheming on how he can mess us up. He'll even have well-meaning people approach you with their comments in order to discourage you. It's important that you use your authority over the devil and his evil spirits and rebuke and bind them; "Whatsoever you bind on earth will be bond in heaven, and what so ever you loose on earth will be loosed in heaven" (Matt. 18:18). So don't wait for the attacks to come; speak to the attacks before they come and cancel the assignment of the enemy. An attack is an act of war, and yes you will experience some level of spiritual warfare in this area, because the flesh is always at war with God. The flesh is really a mind-set. When your fleshly mind-set begins to become challenged regarding this area, that's when the war will began. It began when you picked up this book. But true to any war, when you have the right artillery in your arsenal, it is easier to win the battle. The word of God, prayers, worship, and rebuking and binding up the enemy and his evil spirits are your spiritual arsenal, and the nutritional and physical fitness concepts I have laid out in this book are your natural arsenal.

When I began my own transformation, family and friends alike had all types of things to say. To them, I'm sure it seemed harmless, but those little comments could have been enough to discourage me, if it had not been for God shielding my mind and my heart. Some tried to push food on me, and others made subtle but negative comments about my physique as it changed. I even heard someone quote a scripture about when Paul said the "physical exercise prophets little." It didn't really trouble me, but I sought to understand the context in which Paul was speaking when he made that comment. I later learned from one of the pastors at my church, that what Paul was saying is that compared to the spiritual aspect of our lives, the physical aspect is less important. It is far more important to be concerned about our spiritual health. He didn't mean that it was not important to engage in physical exercise. Ultimately, every Christian should understand that it is the spiritual aspect of our lives that are going to count. That's why it is so important to see even this area of your life on a spiritual level. I had to settle it within myself that as long as I was happy with how I looked and how I ate, that's all that mattered. I stopped expecting those around me to understand the changes I was making and realized I didn't need their approval. So settle with God, and within yourself, that you're just going to do it. The Lord cares about every detail of our lives, and there is no area that he is not concerned about. Praying and asking for God's help, and praising and worshiping him when you want to quit, will allow you to stay focused, while at the same time increasing your fellowship with him, improving the quality of your personal relationship with God.

Eat a balanced diet that contains protein, the right kind of fats, and the right type of carbohydrates (low- to middle-glycemic, that included complex carbohydrates, and the right type of simple sugars, like fruits). All meals should contain a main source of protein, a main source of a carbohydrate (for the most part stay away from meals containing two starches like bread and potatoes in the same meal), and one source of a good fat.

Portion control is important, because healthy food or not, excess calories lead to weight gain and other health problems. Reading and sticking to serving size guidelines will help. If the serving size seems too small, find low-calorie ways to add fullness to the item, like throwing in some fruits and vegetables. Eating five small meals a day every three hours will satisfy better both physically and psychologically.

Drink plenty of water. Don't forget to pay attention to sugar and sodium consumption. It's easy to forget how these two things also play a role in your ability to lose weight, changing your body composition from being more fatty in appearance to being more toned and muscular in appearance, and how well your body otherwise functions.

Engage in cardiovascular training at least three times per week for twenty minutes to forty-five minutes, remembering to focus on intensity, especially if there is very little time. Changes can be made to any cardiovascular program by doing different types like running, biking, swimming, aerobics, praise dancing, etc. The type can be changed on a weekly and daily bases, and so can the intensity. Group cardio can be exciting and fun, and take your mind off of the fact that you are exercising. I encourage you to get a group of friends, do it with your spouse, and get the kids involved as well.

Strength train two to three times per week: This can be achieved with or without dumbbells, barbells, and weight machines. Depending on what you're doing, it can take anywhere from thirty minutes to an hour. You can break it up to do lower body one day and upper body the next (which I think is easiest for the beginner) or do a total body routine. However you break it up, it's important to just do it, and allow the body adequate rest. For example, it's probably not the smartest idea to do the same body part two days in a row. If not careful, this can cause a deterioration of the muscles fibers, causing the muscles not to function as well as they should.

Between cardio and strength training, you can expect to be exercising at least three to five times per week (three times per week if you strength train and do cardio on the same day). Coupled with proper food intake, you can be sure that your level of fitness will increase and you will see bodily changes.

It is important to eat before you work out, especially if you have not eaten in a few hours. It can be something small like a fruit, a shake, some yogurt, or a small energy bar. After the workout, if at all possible, eat within thirty to forty-five minutes of exercising to provide nutrients for the muscles, which at this time are at their peak for absorbing nutrients. I usually have a protein shake (that has at least 25 grams of carbs in it), because liquids are faster to digest and are therefore more quickly absorbed by the body than solid food. Your five meals to six meals can be planned around this, but if they cannot be, don't worry about it—doing this can enhance you results but won't necessarily hinder you.

Use supplements to complement your efforts because they are a non-calorie way to get the nutrients your body needs for the changes you are making.

Eating healthy, being physically active and paying attention to other health-related issues is important. It is important because our bodies are what we present to God as a sacrifice, and because the body is the means by which we physically do what God has spiritually ordained us to do. It's the body that carries out the physical part of our spiritual gifts. Becoming fit for the purpose of doing that which will advance the kingdom of our Lord and savior Jesus Christ and be pleasing to God, will move you beyond the realm of vanity (although there's nothing wrong with wanting to look good), focusing your heart and mind on being fit for the kingdom.

"Beloved, I pray that you may prosper in all things, and be in health, just as your soul prospers (2 John 2:)." May the Lord bless you and keep you in every way—body, soul, and spirit.

About The Author

Weight loss client-turned fitness professional (National Academy of Sports Medicine), physical education teacher (M.S Hofstra University), and minister Pandora Kinard has been in the health and fitness industry for over 13 years.

Within that time, she has introduced lifelong fitness into the lives of people who like herself, thought it to be impossible, and is inspiring the next generation to be active and stay fit.

Her own incredible weight loss journey and path to fitness was featured on channel 7 Eyewitness news (New York City), and in Women's World Magazine. Pandora is also an accomplished fitness writer authoring countless articles on health fitness for various publications.

As a fitness expert and a minister, Pandora has lectured in many churches and other forums about the connection between physical fitness and spirituality, and is a highly regarded and sought after speaker, advisor, and fitness consultant who currently runs her own fitness company (Alpha Omega Fitness in NYC).

Printed in the United States
By Bookmasters